Eye

Manual of Orbital and Lacrimal Surgery

To my sons, Hugh, Michael and George

Manual of Orbital and Lacrimal Surgery

Second edition

Alan A. McNab FRACO, FRACS, FRCOphth

Consultant Ophthalmologist, Royal Victorian Eye and Ear Hospital,
Royal Children's Hospital, Melbourne and Royal Melbourne Hospital,
Australia

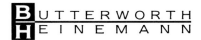

OXFORD BOSTON JOHANNESBURG MELBOURNE NEW DELHI SINGAPORE

Butterworth-Heinemann
Linacre House, Jordan Hill, Oxford OX2 8DP
225 Wildwood Avenue, Woburn, MA 01801-2041
A division of Reed Educational and Professional Publishing Ltd

Ꝟ A member of the Reed Elsevier plc group

First published 1994 by Longman Group UK Limited
Second edition 1998

British Library Cataloguing in Publication Data
A catalogue record for this book is available from the British Library

Library of Congress Cataloguing in Publication Data
A catalogue record for this book is available from the Library of Congress

ISBN 0 7506 3997 0

Data manipulation by David Gregson Associates, Beccles, Suffolk
Printed and bound in Great Britain by The Bath Press plc, Avon

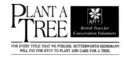

FOR EVERY TITLE THAT WE PUBLISH, BUTTERWORTH-HEINEMANN
WILL PAY FOR BTCV TO PLANT AND CARE FOR A TREE.

Contents

Preface to the second edition

Several additions have been made to the second edition of this text, including chapters on clinical and imaging features of commoner orbital disorders, diagnosis and investigation of lacrimal disease, and the increasingly popular endonasal approach to lacrimal surgery. The aim of the book remains the same however: to serve as a simple practical guide to the surgeon who operates only occasionally on the orbit or lacrimal system. Many ophthalmologists express a fear of orbital surgery. By simplifying the approach to orbital surgery in this manual, it is hoped that when confronted with an unusual and daunting procedure, the occasional orbital surgeon may be more at ease and produce a better outcome for the patient. Many ophthalmologists express a dislike of lacrimal surgery and discourage their patients from undergoing what should be a straightforward operation. By following the simple principles outlined here, mainly aimed at making surgery relatively bloodless and therefore more easily performed, ophthalmologists may find that lacrimal surgery becomes less daunting and more successful. The book may also serve those who are preparing for specialist examinations and may have limited access to the types of procedures outlined here, but who require an understanding of the principles involved.

1998 A.A.M.

Preface to the first edition

This short text is aimed at those who may from time to time operate on the orbit, or who require a knowledge of orbital and lacrimal surgery without the possibility of observing it. Such readers may be remote from the subspecialist care provided by an experienced orbital surgeon, or be preparing for specialist examinations. Other orbital surgeons and other subspecialists whose practice impinges on the orbit may find here one orbital surgeon's distilled methods of interest. This book is by no means intended as a means of learning the difficult task of managing complex orbital diseases, which of course only comes with appropriate training and experience. The emphasis is on those operations which might be considered within the realm of ophthalmologists, but clearly many orbital operations will require the expert help of other specialist surgeons. These methods are beyond the scope of the book.

1994 A.A.M.

1

Surgical anatomy of the orbit and lacrimal system

A good knowledge of orbital and lacrimal anatomy is esential for those intending to operate in the area. This chapter serves as an overview of the suject, and emphasizes those anatomical features of importance to the surgeon. More detailed descriptions will be found in standard anatomical texts.

The bony orbit contains and partly protects the eye and its accessory organs. Its four walls narrow posteriorly towards an apex, which transmits nerves and vessels between the cranial cavity and the orbit. The anterior opening of the orbit is largely filled by the globe and covered by the eyelids, which are separated from the orbit by the orbital septum.

The eyelids

Surgical access to the orbit is often via the eyelid skin or the skin overlying the orbital rim. In the upper eyelid there is a skin fold, the supratarsal fold, which in Caucasians lies ~10 mm above the lashes, and marks the point of insertion of the aponeurosis of the levator palpebrae superioris into the underlying orbicularis oculi muscle fibres. In the lower lid there is often a similar fold, less well-marked and more variable in position. These folds may be used to partially mask scars. The eyebrow will also partially conceal a healed incision.

The eyelid skin is extremely thin and generally devoid of fat. Over the orbital rim, the skin becomes much thicker, especially superiorly, where it more closely resembles the scalp.

Beneath the skin lies the orbicularis oculi muscle, its fibres running circumferentially around the opening of the eyelids and extending beyond the orbital rim. The tarsal plates lie deep to orbicularis and are attached medially to the anterior and posterior lacrimal crests by the medial palpebral ligament. Laterally, they attach to Whitnall's tubercle just inside the lateral orbital rim. In the upper lid, the aponeurosis of the levator muscle divides to attach into the orbicularis muscle fibres and the upper anterior surface of the tarsal plate. The levator aponeurosis

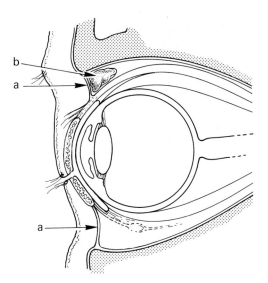

Fig. 1.1. A sagittal section of the orbit.
a = orbital septum;
b = pre-aponeurotic fat pad.

expands medially and laterally as the horns to attach to the orbital rims with the palpebral ligaments. The equivalent structure in the lower lid is the retractor of the lower lid, or the capsulopalpebral head of the inferior rectus muscle.

The orbital septum separates the eyelids from the orbit (Fig. 1.1) and acts as an important barrier to the spread of infection from the lids. It arises from the orbital rim and extends towards the eyelid margins. In the upper lid it fuses with the upper surface of the levator aponeurosis above its insertion into the tarsal plate. In the lower lid it fuses with the retractors a few millimetres below the tarsal plate. Behind the orbital septum lies the orbit proper. In the upper lid the first structure encountered posterior to the septum is the pre-aponeurotic fat pad, which lies in the space between septum and levator aponeurosis. A similar fat pad is found in the lower lid.

The bony orbital walls

Each wall of the orbit has particular relations of importance (Fig. 1.2). The roof of the orbit has the anterior cranial fossa and frontal sinus above. The medial wall has the ethmoid sinuses and posteriorly part of the sphenoid sinus lying medial to it. Below the orbital floor lies the maxillary antrum. The lateral wall has the temporal fossa with the temporalis muscle within it lying lateral to its anterior part. More posteriorly, the lateral wall lies in front of the middle cranial fossa.

The thinnest bone is found in the medial wall of the orbit, separating the ethmoid air cells from the orbit. Anteriorly in the medial wall lies

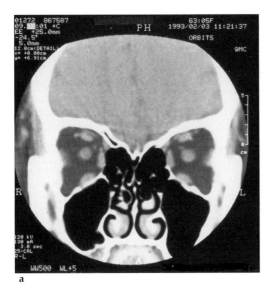
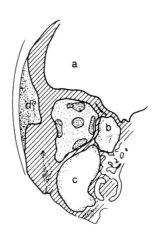

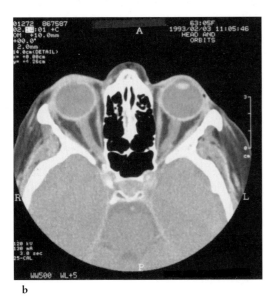
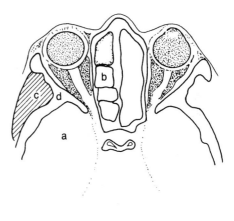

Fig. 1.2 a. Coronal image of the orbit. a = frontal lobe of brain in anterior cranial fossa; b = ethmoid sinuses; c = maxillary antrum; d = temporalis muscle.
b. Axial image of the orbit. a = temporal lobe of the brain in middle cranial fossa; b = ethmoid sinuses; c = temporalis muscle; d = greater wing of sphenoid bone.

the fossa which houses the lacrimal sac, bounded in front by the anterior lacrimal crest and behind by the posterior lacrimal crest. The orbital floor is also very thin, especially medially. The lateral wall has a thinner portion in its middle third, between the orbital rim and the thicker bone of the greater wing of the sphenoid.

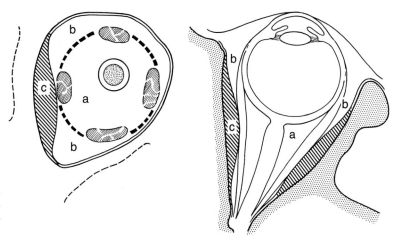

Fig. 1.3. The surgical spaces of the orbit. a = the intraconal space; b = the extraconal space; c = the (potential) extraperiosteal space.

Surgical spaces

The orbit can be divided into three surgical 'spaces' (Fig. 1.3). Between the bone and the periorbita (or periosteum lining the orbit) is the potential subperiosteal space. The extraocular muscles (forming a cone with its apex posteriorly) are partly joined by an intermuscular septum, more marked anteriorly, which divides the orbital contents into an intraconal and an extraconal space.

The subperiosteal space provides surgical access in an easily dissected plane, and may house collections of blood or pus, or other pathological processes. Tumours may be confined to the intra or extraconal space, but the intermuscular 'septum' provides little or no barrier to the spread of tumour, infection or blood except in the young, where (for example) an intraconal haematoma may remain confined without spreading extraconally. The periosteum on the other hand is an important barrier, confining many pathological processes to either of its surfaces.

THE SUBPERIOSTEAL SPACE

This 'space' exists only when surgically created or filled by a pathological process, and follows the contours of the orbital walls. There are a number of structures passing through this space (Fig. 1.4) which are encountered when dissecting in this plane, for example when exenterating the orbit.

To reach the subperiosteal space, the periosteum is incised and elevated over the orbital rim. Around the orbital rim, the periosteum is much more firmly adherent (along the arcus marginalis) than within the orbital walls, where it strips from the bone quite easily.

In elevating the periorbita from the lateral orbital wall, a tenting up of

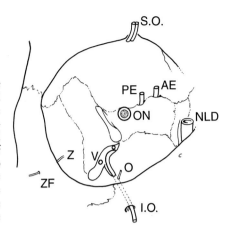

Fig. 1.4. Structures passing through the orbital walls. The roof: SO = supraorbital vessels and nerve. The lateral wall: Z = zygomatic nerve; ZF = zygomatico-facial nerve. The floor: IO = infraorbital vessels and nerve; O = orbital branch of infraorbital artery; V = vein passing into infraorbital fissure. The medial wall: PE = posterior ethmoidal vessels; AE = anterior ethmoidal vessels and nerve; NLD = nasolacrimal duct. Orbital apex: ON = optic nerve.

the periorbita is seen at the site of exit of the zygomatic neurovascular bundle, a variable but short distance inside the rim closer to the floor than the roof. Just posterior and inferior to this will be found the front end of the inferior orbital fissure, with periorbita passing through it with some veins and fat from the orbit to the infratemporal and pterygo-palatine fossas.

Also passing from the inferior orbital fissure into the orbit, but into the floor, is the infraorbital neurovascular bundle; this remains outside the periorbita except for a small branch of the artery (almost invariably found midway back along the floor) which passes upwards, piercing the periorbita. On the medial part of the floor just inside the orbital rim and just lateral to the nasolacrimal duct is the origin of the inferior oblique muscle.

At the junction of the floor and the medial wall, just inside the rim, the nasolacrimal duct pierces the periorbita and passes into the nasolacrimal canal. Where the medial wall meets the roof of the orbit, two (occasionally three) other neurovascular bundles pierce the periorbita. These structures – the anterior and posterior ethmoidal vessels and nerves – serve as a useful landmark for the upper limit of the medial wall when doing a medial wall orbital decompression. The larger anterior ethmoidal bundle is found one-third to half way back from the rim, and the posterior a variable distance behind that, sometimes quite close to the orbital apex.

The orbital roof normally has no structures passing through it but has an important convexity lying anterolaterally, the lacrimal fossa, wherein lies the lacrimal gland. In the superior orbital rim, the supraorbital neurovascular bundle may pass through a canal in the bone and therefore pierce the periorbita anteriorly, but it may also

Fig. 1.5. Structures passing through the superior orbital fissure and optic canal. Z = annulus of Zinn (origin of rectus muscles); ON = optic nerve; OA = ophthalmic artery; L = lacrimal nerve; F = frontal nerve; T = trochlear nerve; V = vein; III^S = superior division of the oculomotor nerve; III^I = inferior division of oculomotor nerve; NC = nasociliary nerve; A = abducens nerve.

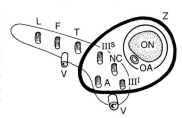

remain within the periorbita as it leaves the orbit via a groove or notch.

At the junction of the roof and lateral walls posteriorly, there lies the superior orbital fissure. This is shorter than the inferior fissure and contains many more structures of importance (Fig. 1.5). The oculomotor nerve in its upper and lower divisions, the trochlear nerve and the abducens nerve, as well as the first division of the trigeminal nerve, all pass through here. Venous connections between the orbit and cavernous sinus are also present.

At the orbital apex, where the roof meets the medial wall, there is the optic foramen. This transmits the optic nerve in its meninges, and the ophthalmic artery.

THE EXTRACONAL SPACE

The most important structure in the extraconal space is the lacrimal gland, which lies in the superotemporal quadrant of the orbit inside the orbital rim, in its own bony lacrimal fossa. The lacrimal gland has two distinct lobes. The larger orbital lobe lies adjacent to the bone of the lacrimal fossa, separated from it by the periorbita, and partly overlies the lateral horn of the levator aponeurosis. It is joined to the smaller palpebral lobe behind the posterior edge of the lateral horn, which therefore partly splits the gland. All the ductules from the orbital lobe pass through the palpebral lobe on their way to the superolateral conjunctival fornix. The blood supply to the gland, via the lacrimal artery, enters the orbital lobe posteriorly.

THE EXTRAOCULAR MUSCLES

The four recti, the superior oblique and levator palpebrae all arise at the apex of the orbit and pass anteriorly as a cone to attach to the globe and lid. The superior oblique has an indirect attachment via the trochlea, which is situated anterosuperiorly inside the orbital rim. The trochlea is firmly attached to the bone here via the periosteum.

The recti and levator receive their innervation from within the muscle cone, with the nerves entering the muscle bellies on the aspect facing into the cone at the junction of the posterior and middle thirds of the muscle. The exceptions are the oblique muscles. The trochlear nerve passes obliquely over the origin of the levator muscle at the orbital apex and enters the belly of the superior oblique on the superior aspect of its posterior third.

The inferior oblique arises at the front of the orbit, from the periorbita, just lateral to the opening of the nasolacrimal canal. It passes laterally and superiorly, piercing the retractors of the lower lid and passing beneath the inferior rectus towards its insertion on the postero-lateral aspect of the globe. It receives innervation from the inferior division of the oculomotor nerve via a long branch passing forwards near the floor of the orbit between the lateral and inferior recti, and enters the muscle near the lateral aspect of the lateral rectus on its bulbar aspect.

THE INTRACONAL SPACE

Within the muscle cone lies orbital fat, the optic nerve and blood vessels and nerves. The ophthalmic artery, entering the orbit with the optic nerve through the optic foramen, breaks up into several branches with inconstant courses. The main artery enters the orbit between the optic nerve and the lateral rectus and usually crosses above the optic nerve to its medial side, passing towards the medial orbital wall. The first and most important branch is the central retinal artery, which arises near the apex of the orbit and runs forwards beneath the optic nerve to pierce its dura about 10 mm behind the globe.

Long and short posterior ciliary nerves and vessels pass forwards within the intraconal space arranged around the optic nerve, but are more numerous on its lateral side. The short ciliary nerves pass from the ciliary ganglion near the orbital apex, between artery and lateral rectus, to the back of the globe.

The lacrimal drainage system

The lacrimal punctae mark the commencement of the lacrimal drainage system (Fig. 1.6). Their openings on the lid margins lead into a 2-mm vertical component of the canaliculus, followed by a horizontal portion 8–10 mm long. The common canaliculus, 1–2 mm in length, leads into the lacrimal sac. It enters the lacrimal sac anteriorly at the internal

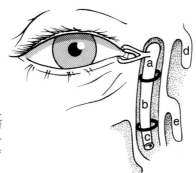

Fig. 1.6. The lacrimal excretory system. a = lacrimal sac; b = intraosseous part of the nasolacrimal duct; c = intramembranous part of nasolacrimal duct; d = middle turbinate; e = inferior turbinate.

common punctum, which is often partially covered by a flap of mucosa known as the valve of Rosenmuller. The lacrimal sac is about 10 mm long vertically, with 3–5 mm of the sac (the fundus) above the common internal punctum. The sac leads into the nasolacrimal duct within the bony nasolacrimal canal, which is 12–15 mm in length. It extends for about 5 mm below the bony canal as an intraepithelial or meatal segment, opening beneath the inferior turbinate in the lateral wall of the nose. A mucosal valve (of Hasner) usually prevents retrogade passage of mucus or air up the duct.

The anterior limb of the medial canthal tendon inserts just anterior to the anterior lacrimal crest. It lies anterior to the lacrimal sac, and a small portion of the sac extends above the upper border of the tendon. The angular vessels usually lie between the skin and orbicularis muscle, on the side of the nose medial to the insertion of the anterior limb of the canthal tendon.

The bony lacrimal fossa (Fig. 1.7) is bounded in front by the anterior lacrimal crest of the frontal process of the maxilla. This crest runs continuously with the inferior orbital rim, but fades superiorly. The posterior lacrimal crest marks the posterior limit of the lacrimal fossa and is formed by the lacrimal bone. The posterior crest continues into the lateral border of the opening of the bony nasolacrimal canal. Running vertically down the lacrimal fossa is the suture line between

Fig. 1.7. The bony lacrimal fossa. a = anterior lacrimal crest; b = posterior lacrimal crest; c = suture line between lacrimal bone and frontal process of maxilla.

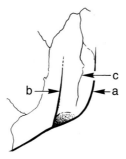

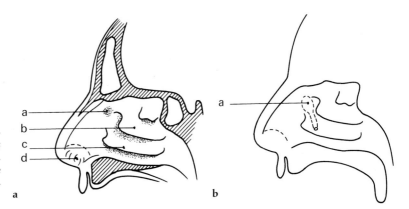

Fig. 1.8 a. Lateral wall of the nose. a = the agger nasi; b = middle turbinate; c = inferior turbinate; d = nasal vestibule. **b** Lateral wall of the nose to show the position of the lacrimal sac and nasolacrimal duct. a = lacrimal sac.

the lacrimal bone and the frontal process of the maxilla, which is usually situated one-half to two-thirds of the way between the anterior and posterior crests. The lacrimal bone behind the suture line is thin, and the bone anterior to the suture line thickens to become thickest at the anterior lacrimal crest.

Knowledge of the anatomy of the lateral wall of the nose is important when performing endonasal lacrimal surgery. The relation of the lacrimal sac and nasolacrimal duct to the lateral nasal wall is illustrated in Fig. 1.8. Whilst there is considerable variation, the lacrimal sac usually lies lateral to a point just in front of the leading edge of the root of the middle turbinate. At this point there is often an elevation or prominence marking the frontal process of the maxilla, called the agger nasi (agger = mound or rampart in Latin). An air cell may lie deep to this, intervening between the nasal mucosa and the lacrimal sac.

Further reading

Bron, A. J. (1997). *Wolff's Anatomy of the Eye and Orbit*, 8th edn. Chapman and Hall.

Duke-Elder, S. (1961). *System of Ophthalmology. Volume 2, The Anatomy of the Visual System.* C V Mosby.

Rootman, J., Stewart, B. and Goldberg, R. A. (1995). Atlas of orbital anatomy. In *Orbital Surgery. A Conceptual Approach* pp. 79–150. Lippincott-Raven.

Whitnall, S. E. (1979). *Anatomy of the Human Orbit and Accessory Organs of Vision* (Facsimile of 1921 edn). Robert E Krieger Publishing.

Zide, B. M. and Jelks, G. W. (1985). *Surgical Anatomy of the Orbit.* Raven Press.

2

Diagnosis and investigation of orbital disease

History and examination

As in any branch of medicine, much can be learned from a thorough history and examination of a patient with orbital disease. Despite the advances represented by computed X-ray tomography (CT scanning) and magnetic resonance imaging (MRI), the radiologist is often not able to provide more than a list of possible diagnoses. The clinician, however, with symptoms and signs plus imaging of the patient, will be able to narrow the possibilities considerably.

HISTORY

Symptoms indicating orbital disease are limited in number:

1. Displacement of the eye (proptosis)
2. Visual disturbance
3. Double vision
4. Pain
5. Swelling
6. A lump
7. Drooping of the upper lid (ptosis)
8. Numbness, or other sensory disturbance.

Each symptom should be analysed carefully in terms of its nature, severity and duration. The duration of symptoms may be the only clue to the nature of a lesion that, radiologically, could be either benign or malignant, with a long duration implying a benign process. The onset of symptoms is equally important − a very sudden onset suggests a vascular event such as a haemorrhage.

In addition to the history of the local disease process, the patient's general medical and surgical history should be obtained. Metastasis to the orbit is not uncommon, and thyroid eye disease is the commonest cause of proptosis (exophthalmos).

EXAMINATION

The examination should be both local and general, and the local examination should include the following.

Assessment of visual function

1. Visual acuity

2. Visual fields

3. Colour vision

4. Pupil function (afferent defects).

Position of the globe

1. Its anteroposterior position in relation to the lateral orbital rim or other fixed point, and in relation to the other globe. This is measured with an exophthalmometer, or a rough estimate may be made by looking down on the patient's eyes from above and behind.

2. Any horizontal or vertical shift from the normal position. This is determined with reference to the other eye, by using a clear plastic ruler and measuring from the midline to the medial or lateral limbus. The patient's other eye is covered to overcome any manifest deviation of the globe. Any vertical shift is measured by placing the ruler horizontally across the eyes and looking for displacement of the eye compared to its fellow.

If the globe is displaced forwards (proptosed) without vertical or horizontal displacement, this is termed axial proptosis, and the disease process is either intraconal or affecting the orbital structures in a symmetrical way (such as in thyroid eye disease).

Vertical and horizontal deviation occurs usually by a mass pushing the globe away; so, for example, a mass in the lacrimal gland causes downwards and medial displacement of the globe.

Occasionally, a disease process may cause enophthalmos (metastatic breast carcinoma is an example). Pseudoproptosis may occur, with gross facial asymmetry or disparity in the size of the globes (unilateral axial myopia or an exceptionally small eye).

The upper cranial nerves
This includes assessing eye movements which may be affected by either nerve damage, muscle damage or mechanical factors. Facial and ocular

sensation and facial nerve and muscle function are examined. Loss of sensation in the area of distribution of one of the sensory nerves is an important sign, and may indicate a malignant process.

Ocular examination

External ocular examination (including the lids and conjunctival fornices), slit lamp examination and fundal examination are all important. The eye is observed to see if there is any variation in its position with the valsalva manoeuvre, or in time with the pulse (pulsatile proptosis), as may occur with defects in the orbital roof or posterolateral wall (transmitted brain pulsation) or with arteriovenous malformations.

Palpation of the orbit

The orbit is systematically palpated for the presence of any masses. All quadrants are felt with a finger, using the little finger if there is not much space between the globe and the orbital rim. The bony margins should also be palpated.

Examination of contiguous structures

The temporal fossa (for fullness from sphenoidal wing meningioma), face and nasal passages should be examined. An essential part of the examination is palpation of the regional lymph nodes (pre-auricular, submandibular and cervical).

General examination

Features of thyroid disease should be sought. A full examination may reveal systemic disease of which the orbital disease is only a component (e.g. lymphoma, metastatic breast carcinoma).

Investigations

Where CT scanning facilities exist, this will be the prime form of investigation of orbital disease. Plain X-ray of the orbit may provide useful information, but is redundant in the presence of good CT scanning.

CT SCANNING

CT scanning has revolutionized the investigation of orbital disease.

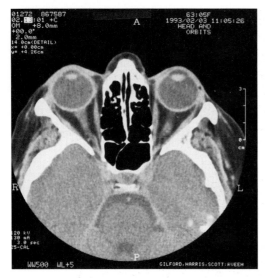

Fig. 2.1. Axial CT scan of the orbits.

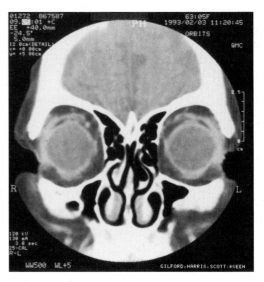

Fig. 2.2. Coronal CT scan of the orbits through the globe.

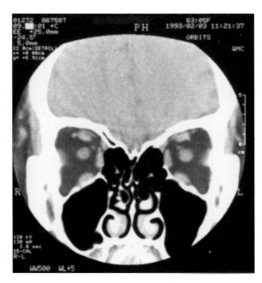

Fig. 2.3. Coronal CT scan of the orbits through the middle third.

However, it is no substitute for a careful and thorough history and examination, which are merely complemented by the CT scan.

When ordering CT scans, both axial and coronal images should be obtained if possible (Figs 2.1–2.3). Coronal images may give information not readily appreciated on axial images, such as the relationship of an intraconal mass to the optic nerve. Most radiologists will provide both pre- and post-contrast studies, and contrast enhancement may be useful in differentiating some lesions.

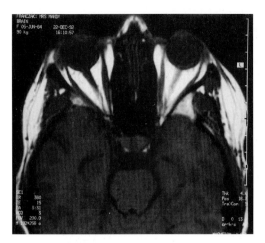

Fig. 2.4. Axial MRI of the orbits.

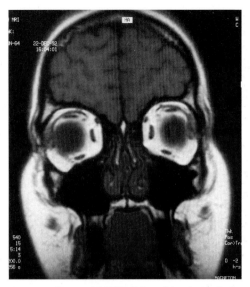

Fig. 2.5. Coronal MRI of the orbits through the globe

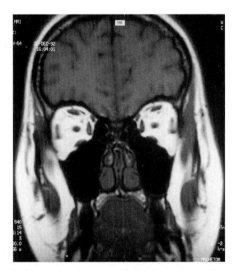

Fig. 2.6. Coronal MRI of the orbits through the middle third.

Bone window settings of CT scans can provide information on the orbital walls which may be missed on soft tissue settings. Subtle bone erosion, as may occur with carcinomas, is an example.

MAGNETIC RESONANCE IMAGING

This is an increasingly available investigation, which may supplement CT scanning. It is particularly good at delineating soft tissues, but does not show bone (Figs 2.4–2.6). Certain tumours may be more readily seen in their full extent using MRI, especially with the use of contrast agents. The other principal advantage of MRI is that images may be made in any plane (sagittal, axial, coronal or others). Newer software programs allow images to be constructed of the vascular channels (magnetic resonance angiography or MRA), and a similar function is available on some CT scanners.

OTHER INVESTIGATIONS

Occasionally, other investigations may be of use in the investigation of orbital disease. These include ultrasonography and angiography, which can now be performed with MRI without the need for arterial catheterization.

Ultrasonography generally provides little more than can be obtained from a good CT scan, although internal reflectivity within certain tumours may occasionally help differentiate those that appear identical on CT. The addition of Doppler to the ultrasound may indicate blood flow and its direction.

Further reading

De Potter, P., Shields, J. A. and Shields, C. L. (1995). *MRI of the Eye and Orbit.* J B Lippincott.
Krohel, G. B., Stewart, W. B. and Chavis, R. M. (1981). *Orbital Disease, a Practical Approach.* Grune and Stratton.
Rootman, J. (1988). *Diseases of the Orbit.* J B Lippincott.

3

Commoner orbital disorders

Almost any pathological process may affect the orbit. Some are much more common than others, and published lists of diagnoses from orbital centres give an indication of the relative frequency of orbital disease processes. Most would agree that the commonest orbital disorder is thyroid orbitopathy (also called Graves' ophthalmopathy, thyroid eye disease, etc.). Other diagnoses differ in their frequency, depending on referral patterns, geography, population factors and other biases.

A useful grouping of orbital disorders can be made as follows:

1. Congenital/structural
2. Inflammatory
3. Vascular
4. Neoplastic
5. Degenerative/deposits
6. Traumatic.

Some of the more common disorders within each of these groups are described below. Rarer diseases are generally not discussed, unless they are an important differential diagnosis. It is not intended to provide detailed descriptions; those are beyond the scope of this text, and readers are referred to more comprehensive texts (see Further reading).

Congenital/structural

1. Dermoid cyst
2. Microphthalmos with cyst
3. Encephalocoele
4. Craniofacial dysostoses.

DERMOID CYST

A dermoid cyst is a developmental lesion classified as a choristoma (proliferation of normal tissue in an abnormal position). The cyst is lined

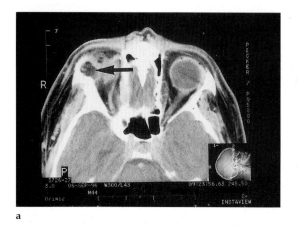

a

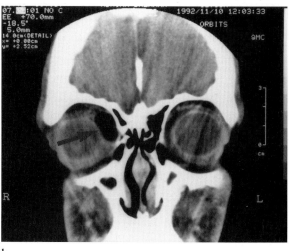

b

Fig. 3.1 a. Axial CT of a right temporal orbital dermoid cyst (arrow). The cyst contents are of low density, and there is a bony defect in the lateral orbital rim with recent spontaneous cyst rupture causing inflammation.
b. Coronal CT of a right medial orbital dermoid cyst (arrow), with characteristic low density contents.

by epithelium derived from surface ectoderm (skin), with skin appendages such as hair follicles and associated glandular structures. Cysts gradually enlarge and may leak their contents into surrounding tissues, exciting an inflammatory response. If not removed completely, a draining sinus may result. They occur most commonly near the surface in relation to the superolateral orbital rim (external angular dermoid), and in the superomedial anterior orbit. External angular dermoids present early in life, and medial dermoids also usually occur in childhood. Deeper dermoids may be lateral or medial (Fig. 3.1a, b), rarely appearing elsewhere in the orbit, and often present later in life with mass effect or with episodes of inflammation due to leakage. There may be associated defects in the bone, sometimes with extensions of the cyst into the temporal fossa. Some medial dermoids may have a conjunctival lining, and some deep, late presenting cysts may be epidermoids, lacking the adnexal structures of a dermoid.

MICROPHTHALMOS WITH CYST

Some microphthalmic eyes have associated cysts connected to the rudimentary globe or optic nerve. These may be large and are sometimes connected to the subarachnoid space. If not too large, they may be left to promote orbital growth.

ORBITAL ENCEPHALOCOELE

These are rare and usually occur medially or on the midline, where they may cause wide separation of the orbits (hypertelorism). Medially, they are an important differential diagnosis for congenital dilatation of the lacrimal sac (dacryocoele or dacryops).

CRANIOFACIAL DYSOSTOSES

This heterogeneous group of congenital anomalies includes Crouzon's disease. They share several features including shallow orbits causing relative proptosis, which may be severe and result in corneal exposure. Surgical treatment is the domain of specialist craniofacial teams. Other related disorders include Treacher Collins syndrome and the hemifacial microsomias/Goldenhar's syndrome complex, which may present with ocular surface solid dermoids at the limbus or on the superolateral globe (dermolipoma).

Inflammatory

1. Thyroid orbitopathy
2. Orbital cellulitis
3. Idiopathic orbital inflammation
4. Specific inflammatory orbital disorders.

THYROID ORBITOPATHY

Thyroid orbitopathy is the commonest single disease entity affecting the orbit. It is an immune-mediated inflammatory process occurring in association with thyroid dysfunction, usually in the form of thyrotoxic goitre (Graves' disease). The inflammatory process is centred on the extraocular muscles and orbital connective tissue, and also includes the lacrimal gland in some cases. In addition to infiltration with inflammatory cells, there is increased volume of tissues due to accumulation of oedema and mucopolysaccharides, as well as fibrosis and vascular congestion. There is a broad spectrum of clinical features, but most patients are mildly affected with only a small minority developing sight-threatening disease. Whilst the disease process tends to run a course of active inflammation over months to years, the orbit is permanently altered by the long-term sequelae of this process.

A number of attempts have been made to classify stages and degrees

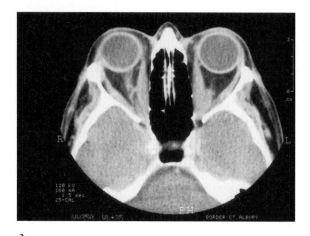

a

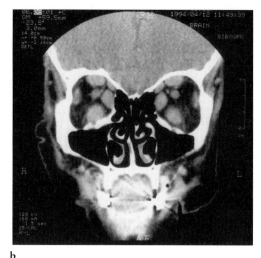

b

Fig. 3.2 a. Axial CT of a patient with severe thyroid orbitopathy. There is a fusiform enlargement of the medial and lateral recti with orbital apical crowding, causing optic neuropathy.
b. Coronal CT through the mid-orbits shows enlargement of the extra-ocular muscles.

of severity of thyroid orbitopathy, but none has been universally accepted. The following clinical features occur to varying degrees, with the later features seen generally in more severe cases.

1. Ocular discomfort, injection, watering

2. Eyelid retraction, lagophthalmos

3. Eyelid and conjunctival oedema and orbital fat protrusion

4. Proptosis (exophthalmos)

5. Extraocular muscle restriction

6. Corneal exposure/ulceration

7. Optic neuropathy.

Patients may progress quite rapidly from mild to moderate or severe disease, but once stable they tend not to change much over time as the permanent sequelae of the inflammatory process set in. The clinical features may be quite asymmetric with apparently unilateral cases sometimes seen, but generally some signs, either clinical or imaging, are seen on the opposite side.

The diagnosis is usually made clinically, in the presence of abnormal thyroid function tests or antibody studies, and with the aid of changes seen on orbital CT (Fig. 3.2a, b) or MRI scans. Some patients present without thyroid dysfunction, and a few may be hypothyroid. Most euthyroid patients will develop thyroid dysfunction within two years.

CT scans usually demonstrate fusiform enlargement of one or more extraocular muscles (Fig. 3.2a, b), increased volume and density of orbital fat, lacrimal gland enlargement and venous engorgement, often seen as an enlarged superior ophthalmic vein. Patients with optic neuropathy (manifest as decreased acuity, field defects and abnormal colour vision) will show enlargement of extraocular muscles, crowding the orbital apex and compressing the optic nerve (Fig. 3.2a).

Current therapy may involve:

1. Symptomatic measures – ocular lubricants, elevation of the head at night
2. Immune modulation – corticosteroids and other immune therapies
3. Orbital irradiation
4. Surgery – orbital decompression, extraocular muscle surgery, eyelid surgery.

Surgery (other than orbital decompression for optic neuropathy) is best performed when the disease has stabilized.

ORBITAL CELLULITIS

This is covered in Chapter 9.

IDIOPATHIC ORBITAL INFLAMMATION

This process, previously referred to by the unsatisfactory term of orbital pseudotumour, may affect any orbital tissue and may be acute or chronic. When largely confined to one structure, it may be specified by such terms as orbital myositis, scleritis, or nonspecific dacryoadenitis (if not due to a specific organism or disease process). In acute or subacute forms, features of inflammation are seen, usually with pain. Other signs and symptoms are determined by the structures affected. If a biopsy can be obtained safely, it is preferable to do this rather than treat such patients speculatively with corticosteroids, as many other disease processes and other specific inflammatory processes may mimic 'pseudotumour'. Chronic forms of the disease do occur, and some of these have fibrosis as their predominating feature (sclerosing idiopathic inflammation). These respond poorly to treatment.

SPECIFIC INFLAMMATORY ORBITAL DISORDERS

Sarcoidosis may affect orbital tissues, most commonly the lacrimal gland, and Sjögren's syndrome may also manifest with lacrimal gland inflammation. Wegener's granulomatosis may have orbital involvement, often in association with paranasal sinus disease.

Vascular

1. Capillary haemangioma
2. Cavernous haemangioma
3. Venous anomalies/lymphangioma
4. Arteriovenous malformations and fistulae
5. Cholesterol granuloma.

CAPILLARY HAEMANGIOMA

Capillary haemangiomas are tumours composed of proliferating endothelially-lined vessels that appear in the first weeks of life, grow for a year or so, and then gradually involute over several years. On the skin they have a characteristic strawberry appearance. In the eyelids, their importance lies in their ability to cause amblyopia by visual deprivation, or induction of astigmatism through globe compression. Orbital capillary haemangiomas may or may not have a cutaneous component, and may also compress the globe or cause strabismus or optic nerve compression. If sight-threatening, they may be treated by local injection of corticosteroids, systemic steroids, a course of subcutaneous interferon, or, if circumscribed, surgical excision may be offered. Treatment must be balanced by the natural history of involution.

CAVERNOUS HAEMANGIOMAS

Cavernous haemangiomas are well circumscribed vascular tumours composed of dilated, blood-filled channels, with very low blood flow. They are more common in middle-aged women and can occur anywhere in the orbit, but are commonest in the intraconal space, lateral to the optic nerve (Fig. 3.3). They may be discovered incidentally when patients are scanned for unrelated symptoms, and in these circumstances may be observed, often not changing significantly over many years. If symptomatic or threatening vision, they may be removed, and do not recur. Cavernous haemangiomas are the classical indication for a lateral orbitotomy.

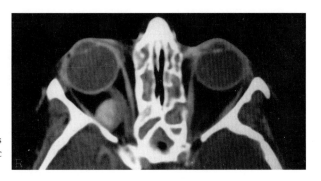

Fig. 3.3. Axial CT shows a cavernous haemangioma lateral to the right optic nerve.

VENOUS ANOMALIES/LYMPHANGIOMA

There is a spectrum of orbital vascular malformations ranging from purely venous (with obvious connections to the venous circulation) to others with characteristics more in keeping with lymphatic malformations (with little or no connection to the circulation). These latter lesions tend to be anterior or conjunctival. A wide variety exists between these extremes. Lesions may be part of a more widespread facial or cranial vascular malformation. Those with obvious connections to the venous circulation may dilate with raised venous pressure, and some bleed spontaneously, and may form 'blood cysts'. They tend to infiltrate normal structures, making surgical excision difficult.

ARTERIOVENOUS MALFORMATIONS AND FISTULAE

True orbital arteriovenous malformations are rare. Secondary involvement of the orbital circulation by arteriovenous fistulae of the cavernous sinus (carotid–cavernous fistulae) are commoner, and may be traumatic or spontaneous, low- or high-flow. Fistulae from the intracavernous carotid artery are usually traumatic and high-flow. Spontaneous fistulae often involve meningeal branches of the internal or external carotid circulation. The orbital signs are due to arterial pressure blood being shunted via the ophthalmic veins into the orbit, causing proptosis, vascular engorgement, motility disturbance, retinal ischaemia and raised intraocular pressure. Treatment, if required, is usually by interventional radiological techniques. The fistulae may be occluded by endovascular techniques, using arterial or venous access. Occasionally, access via the superior ophthalmic vein may be useful.

CHOLESTEROL GRANULOMA

Cholesterol granulomas characteristically occur in the region of the lacrimal gland fossa in the frontal bone. They may be due to

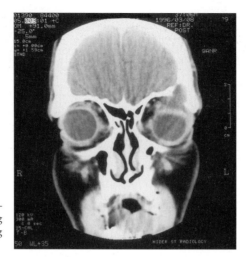

Fig. 3.4. Coronal CT of a left orbito-frontal cholesterol granuloma displacing and compressing the globe and eroding the frontal bone.

haemorrhage occurring in the diploë of the bone, expanding and causing resorption of bone, and extension into the extraperiosteal space of the orbit (Fig. 3.4) or even extradurally in the anterior cranial fossa. Some patients give a history of trauma. There is a granulomatous response centred on cholesterol crystals and other blood breakdown products. The lesion is simply treated by drainage and curettage.

Neoplastic

1. Primary
   a. Lacrimal gland
   b. Neurogenic
   c. Mesenchymal
   d. Lymphocytic/leukaemic/histiocytic
2. Secondary
   a. Metastatic
   b. Direct spread from adjacent structures.

PRIMARY TUMOURS

Lacrimal gland

Lacrimal gland neoplasms are similar in their spectrum to salivary gland tumours. The epithelial tumours may be benign (pleomorphic adenoma) or malignant. Lymphocytic tumours may also occur within the lacrimal gland.

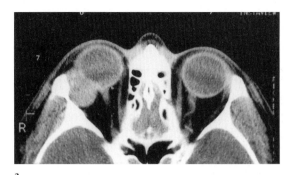
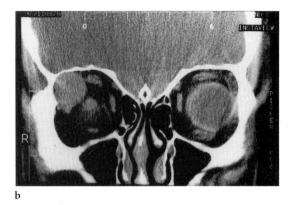

a

b

Fig. 3.5 a. Axial CT of a right pleomorphic adenoma of the lacrimal gland. The mass is well circumscribed and flattens the adjacent globe, and there is remodelling of overlying bone.
b. Coronal CT of a right pleomorphic adenoma which has caused smooth remodelling of the overlying bone.

Pleomorphic adenomas are slow growing benign tumours that may become malignant after many years, and may recur as an infiltrative tumour if not entirely removed within their pseudocapsule. The typical patient presents with slowly progressive, painless proptosis with inferior and medial displacement of the globe. When palpated, these tumours feel firm to hard. CT scans show a well circumscribed lesion of the lacrimal fossa, which is often remoulded, and flattening of the adjacent globe (Fig. 3.5a, b). Once diagnosed clinically and radiologically, they should be removed intact via a lateral orbitotomy (see Chapter 5).

A range of malignant neoplasms occurs within the lacrimal gland, but the commonest is the adenoidcystic carcinoma. The typical history is shorter than a year, with proptosis and pain. On CT scan the tumour may be deceptively well circumscribed, but often a tail of tumour extends towards the superior orbital fissure (Fig. 3.6), and the adjacent

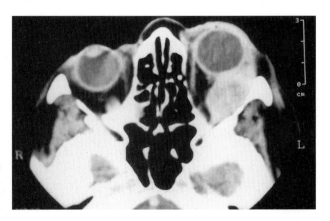

Fig. 3.6. Axial CT of an adenoidcystic carcinoma of the left lacrimal gland. Although apparently well circumscribed, tumour extends towards the orbital apex.

bone is irregularly eroded. These tumours have a propensity to spread along nerves. The optimum management is debated. Very few, if any, are cured, so the place of radical surgery (orbitectomy or extended exenteration) is probably limited and most specialists recommend macroscopic removal of the tumour followed by radiotherapy. Some patients with adenoidcystic carcinoma live for many years with local and distant disease before finally succumbing.

Other malignant lacrimal gland neoplasms include the malignant mixed tumour (a transformed pleomorphic adenoma), adenocarcinoma and mucoepidermoid carcinoma. If a malignant neoplasm is suspected, a biopsy should be obtained via a trans-septal anterior orbitotomy. Once confirmed the options are then a limited resection and radiotherapy, or radical excision (orbitectomy) and free vascularized flap repair with or without radiotherapy.

Neurogenic

Neurogenic orbital tumours include optic nerve meningioma and glioma, neurilemmoma or schwannoma, neurofibroma and plexiform neuroma.

Primary optic nerve meningiomas (Fig. 3.7) occur more commonly in women, and tend to be slow growing. In younger patients, there may be a more aggressive growth pattern with earlier intracranial involvement. Patients present with painless gradual visual loss, mild axial proptosis and optic disc swelling or atrophy, sometimes with shunt vessels. Treatment is debated. Surgical excision involves removal of the entire optic nerve and sheath from the chiasm to the globe and may be offered to younger patients, but this of course means loss of vision in that eye. Radiotherapy may offer some benefits, especially if given by radiosurgical techniques where high doses can be delivered to a small

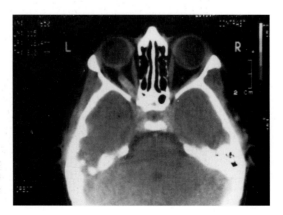

Fig. 3.7. Axial CT of a primary optic nerve sheath meningioma. There is cylindrical enlargement of most of the orbital optic nerve.

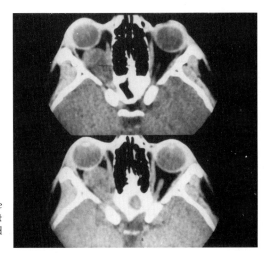

Fig. 3.8. Axial CT of an optic nerve glioma. There is fusiform enlargement of the optic nerve and an enlarged optic canal.

area with reduced effect on surrounding structures. In older patients, simple observation and sequential contrast MRI looking for intracranial extension may be appropriate.

Optic nerve glioma (Fig. 3.8) occurs usually in the first two decades, and more frequently in patients with neurofibromatosis type 1 (NF1). It tends to be slow growing, especially in NF1, but may involve the optic chiasm or contralateral optic nerve. Reasonable visual function may be preserved for long periods with the more indolent gliomas. If a glioma is confined to the optic nerve and is apparently growing, surgical excision may be offered, requiring complete removal of the nerve from the chiasm to the globe via a frontal cranio-orbitotomy.

Neurilemmomas (schwannomas) are benign lesions arising from nerves anywhere within the orbit. They are firm, well circumscribed and smooth (Fig. 3.9), sometimes with macroscopic cystic areas within

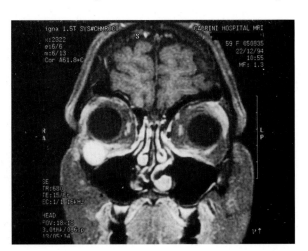

Fig. 3.9. An axial T1 weighted MRI (with contrast) of a neurilemmoma (schwannoma) in the inferior right orbit.

them. They may extend along affected nerves through the superior orbital fissure. Neurofibromas may be isolated or occur as part of neurofibromatosis. A plexiform neuroma is pathognomonic of NF1 and typically occurs in the superolateral orbit, with thickening of the eyelid, enlargement of the orbit and pigmentary changes of the overlying skin. Plexiform neuromas infiltrate normal structures, and although they may be debulked, are not curable. Malignant peripheral nerve tumours are rare.

Mesenchymal

The most important mesenchymal tumour is rhabdomyosarcoma, a childhood tumour, which may present with rapid growth, sometimes mimicking an inflammatory process. Urgent biopsy should be sought, and prognosis for tumours confined to the orbit is good following treatment with chemotherapy and radiotherapy.

Other sarcomas of the orbit are rare, but one mesenchymal tumour that is seen with some regularity is the fibrous histiocytoma, which may behave benignly or aggressively. They tend to be well circumscribed, smooth tumours.

Primary tumours of the orbital bones are uncommon, and include fibrous dysplasia, osteoma, ossifying fibroma and aneurysmal bone cyst. Malignant bone tumours of the orbit are even rarer.

Lymphocytic/histiocytic/leukaemic

Lymphoma is one of the commonest tumours of the orbit. Most tend to be relatively low grade B-cell tumours, and occur in older patients as painless infiltrative lesions of the anterior orbit. Involvement of the orbit may occur with known lymphoma, or as an apparently isolated extranodal manifestation. Some of these patients will have lymphoma elsewhere when investigated, and if systemic work-up is negative, many will develop disease elsewhere over time. Some orbital lymphocytic proliferations are not clearly lymphomatous, and these may be reactive or indeterminate in nature. Again, some of these patients will ultimately develop lymphoma, either locally or elsewhere. On CT scan, lymphocytic lesions tend to infiltrate and obscure tissues, moulding to the globe rather than indenting it (Fig. 3.10). If suspected clinically, a biopsy should be handled in such a way as to give maximum information by consulting with the pathologist. This will usually mean providing fresh tissue.

The most important histiocytic lesion of the orbit is Langerhans' cell histiocytosis, previously known as eosinophilic granuloma. These

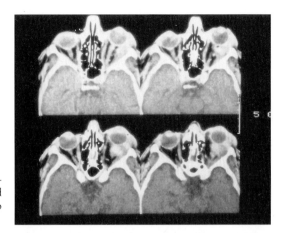

Fig. 3.10. Axial CT scans of a lymphoma centred on the lacrimal gland but extending around and moulding to the globe.

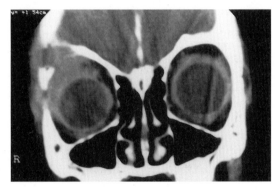

Fig. 3.11. Coronal CT scan of a child with Langerhans' cell histocytosis (eosinophilic granuloma) of the right orbit causing irregular bone destruction of the frontal bone.

lesions typically occur in childhood, centred on the bone of the lacrimal fossa, often with extensive bone erosion (Fig. 3.11). They are often isolated (monostotic), but systemic work-up is mandatory. Treatment varies from curettage through corticosteroids to radiotherapy or chemotherapy.

Leukaemic infiltrates of the orbit may occur in many forms of leukaemia, but the commonest is the granulocytic sarcoma or chloroma, a form of chronic granulocytic leukaemia.

Plasma cell tumours may affect the orbit or orbital bones as solitary plasmacytomas or as part of multiple myeloma.

SECONDARY TUMOURS

Metastases

Metastasis of solid tumours to the orbit is not uncommon. The breast is the most common primary site, and some of these patients will present with a characteristic picture of enophthalmos and restricted motility due to infiltration of the orbit by fibrosing (scirrhous) metastatic breast carcinoma. Other tumours which regularly metastasize to the orbit are those of the lung, prostate, kidney, thyroid and gastrointestinal tract. Prostatic carcinoma may metastasize to orbital bones, with lytic or sclerotic bone changes. In infants and young children, neuroblastoma is a common cause of orbital metastasis, which may be haemorrhagic.

Direct spread from adjacent structures

Direct involvement of the orbit by tumours arising in adjacent structures is common, and is probably the commonest indication for orbital exenteration, usually as part of a wider cancer operation. The potential sites include the eye (retinoblastoma and uveal melanoma), the eyelids (basal and squamous cell carcinoma), the conjunctiva (melanoma and squamous cell carcinoma), the paranasal sinuses, the nose and nasopharynx, and the cranial cavity (most commonly sphenoidal or frontal meningioma).

Eyelid or facial cutaneous tumours may invade the orbit directly or along nerves; this latter feature is seen most commonly with cutaneous squamous cell carcinoma of the face. Basal cell carcinoma has a tendency to spread along periosteal planes, especially from the medial or lateral canthus. Every attempt should be made to ascertain the extent of tumour before embarking on radical surgery.

Degenerative/deposits

This rare group of entities includes progressive hemifacial atrophy (Parry Romberg syndrome), which may present with increasing enophthalmos, and orbital amyloidosis.

Traumatic

Orbital fractures and foreign bodies are dealt with in Chapters 8 and 9. One aspect of orbital trauma worth mentioning here is traumatic orbital haemorrhage, with raised orbital tension causing optic nerve dysfunction or diminished retinal circulation (see Chapter 8). The haemorrhage may be also be iatrogenic, resulting from orbital injection, orbital surgery or surgery on adjacent structures.

Further reading

Henderson, J. W. (1994). *Orbital Tumors,* 3rd edn. Raven Press.
Jones, I. S. and Jakobiec, F. A. (1979). *Diseases of the Orbit.* Harper and Row.
Rootman, J. (1988). *Diseases of the Orbit.* J B Lippincott.
Spencer, W. H. (1996). *Ophthalmic Pathology,* 4th edn. W B Saunders.

4

Orbital tumour surgery

For a patient with an orbital tumour, the following interrelated questions summarize the steps in formulating a surgical plan.

1. What is the site of the lesion?

2. What is the most likely diagnosis?

3. Is an excisional biopsy or incisional biopsy preferred?

4. What is the best surgical approach to the lesion?

Choice of operation

The mere presence of an orbital tumour does not necessitate surgery, and certain tumours may best be left untreated, for example primary optic nerve sheath meningiomas in the elderly. Occasionally, a tumour may be found incidentally when a CT scan is performed for other reasons. The most common of these is an asymptomatic cavernous haemangioma, where there is no indication to operate unless the patient develops symptoms or there is documented growth with the potential for causing serious symptoms.

Usually, a patient presents with symptoms, is examined and investigated, and is found to have a lesion for which the clinician can offer a shortlist of likely diagnoses. The decision then is whether to remove the whole lesion (an excisional biopsy), or to obtain a representative biopsy (incisional biopsy). This decision depends on the most likely diagnosis.

If a lesion is thought to be inflammatory, a lymphoma or some other infiltrative lesion, then an incisional biopsy is appropriate. Similarly, if the lesion is likely to be malignant, an incisional biopsy is planned to make a tissue diagnosis so that a further plan of action can then be made. This may mean radical surgery (orbital exenteration), radiotherapy or chemotherapy, or a combination of these.

For benign, circumscribed lesions such as cavernous haemangiomas, neurilemmomas and dermoid cysts, complete excision is the treatment of choice. Indeed, incisional biopsy or incomplete excision of a dermoid or epidermoid may cause the severe complications of recurrent inflammation, scarring and fistula formation.

A special case is the group of lacrimal gland tumours. If the clinical diagnosis is benign pleomorphic adenoma, then an excisional biopsy without tumour cell spillage is essential. This almost always means a lateral orbitotomy. If the lesion is thought to be inflammatory, lymphoma or carcinoma, then an incisional biopsy via a direct trans-septal route is preferred.

General guidelines for orbital tumour surgery

The following principles apply to any type of orbital tumour surgery:

1. Communicate with the pathologist before the case to determine the preferred method of specimen delivery (fresh or formalinized, etc.). This will depend on the likely diagnosis.

2. Use good illumination and sufficient magnification to see anatomical detail. This may mean a headlight with loupes or an operating microscope, or simply operating room lights.

3. Maintain meticulous haemostasis. This simplifies dissection and identification of pathological tissues. Certain lesions that appear obvious on a CT scan as a marked change may be difficult to differentiate from normal orbital fat or even lacrimal gland if bathed in blood.

4. Use blunt dissection within the orbit. This reduces the risk of damage to normal structures.

5. Repalpate any mass as dissection proceeds, to determine its proximity and relationship to other palpable structures — for example, the globe, optic nerve, trochlea and superior oblique tendon.

6. Handle any pathological specimens very gently, as crushing and distortion may render the specimen useless.

Anterior orbitotomy

1. Trans-septal
2. Transconjunctival
3. Extraperiosteal.

TRANS-SEPTAL ANTERIOR ORBITOTOMY

Principle

A direct approach through the eyelid and orbital septum is made to a lesion to be removed or biopsied.

Indications

1. Planned incisional biopsy of any lesion in the anterior half of the orbit, including lacrimal gland biopsies.

2. Planned excisional biopsy of selected lesions in the anterior half of the orbit. Such lesions include anteriorly placed cavernous haemangiomas, dermoids (but not those placed laterally with an extension through the lateral orbital wall) and neurofibromas, but specifically exclude pleomorphic adenomas of the lacrimal gland, except for the rare cases confined to the palpebral lobe.

Method

1. If general anaesthesia is used, palpate the orbit again. Additional information may be obtained which was not apparent whilst the patient was awake.

2. Mark the incision with a pen (Fig. 4.1), if possible in a natural skin fold (upper lid fold, for example). However, if a malignant lesion is suspected, mark a direct incision over the mass in the direction of the orbicularis fibres.

3. Local anaesthetic may be used for biopsies of relatively superficial lesions or excision of small anteriorly placed masses.

4. Incise the skin with a scalpel.

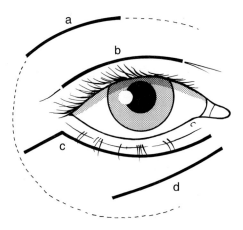

Fig. 4.1. Incisions for anterior transseptal orbitotomy. a = brow incision; b = skin-crease incision; c = subciliary incision; d = lower lid crease incision.

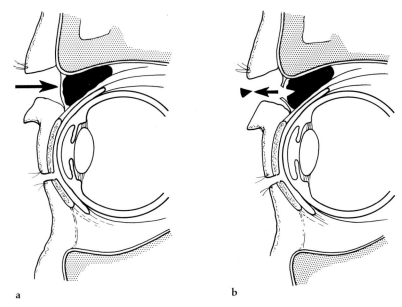

Fig. 4.2 a. Anterior trans-septal orbit-otomy. Skin and orbicularis opened. Arrow at point of entry through orbital septum.
b. Biopsy of an anterior extraconal mass.

a   b

5. Buttonhole the orbicularis, and open the muscle in the direction of its fibres with blunt scissors.

6. Open the orbital septum with blunt scissors (Fig. 4.2a).

7. Expose the lesion by blunt dissection.

8. If a simple incisional biopsy is required, gently hold the tumour by its surface with fine-toothed forceps, and use a scalpel to obtain a representative biopsy (Fig. 4.2b). Do not crush the specimen.

9. If a complete excision is planned, dissect the lesion from surrounding structures and remove the lump intact if possible.

10. Obtain haemostasis. If bleeding continues, place a fine flexible drain (e.g. glove rubber) in the wound, and suture it to the wound edges.

11. Close the orbicularis with several 6/0 plain catgut sutures.

12. Close the skin with a subcuticular 6/0 nylon suture, passing around the drain tube if present, and fixing the ends to the skin with tape (Fig. 4.3). After removal of the drain tube (usually 24 hours), tighten the subcuticular stitch to completely close the wound.

TRANSCONJUNCTIVAL ANTERIOR ORBITOTOMY

Principle

An approach to a lesion to be removed or biopsied is made via the conjunctiva.

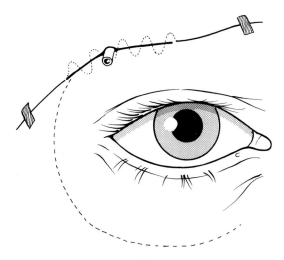

Fig. 4.3. Wound closure with drain tube.

Indications

1. Any lesion visible subconjunctivally which is to have an incisional biopsy (e.g. lymphoma).

2. Anteriorly placed intraconal lesions which are to be biopsied only.

3. Anterior intraconal lesions in children.

4. Unusual tumours presenting subconjunctivally.

5. Approach to the optic nerve for optic nerve sheath fenestration or debulking of a glioma.

6. Lacrimal gland biopsies should NOT be performed transconjunctivally, as the lacrimal ductules will be damaged. Lacrimal gland biopsies (orbital lobe) should be done trans-septally.

Method

1. Visible subconjunctival lesions for biopsy

    a. Incise the conjunctiva directly over the lesion by elevating it with forceps and cutting with scissors.

    b. Expose the lesion by retracting the conjunctiva.

    c. Carefully obtain biopsy material (this will be quite friable in cases of lymphoma).

    d. The conjunctiva may be left open if bleeding is difficult to control, otherwise close it with fine interrupted catgut sutures.

2. Intraconal or optic nerve lesions or nerve sheath fenestration. A medial approach will be described but the principle is the same for a lateral approach.

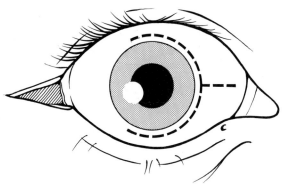

Fig. 4.4. Transconjunctival medial orbitotomy. Line of incisions and lateral canthotomy.

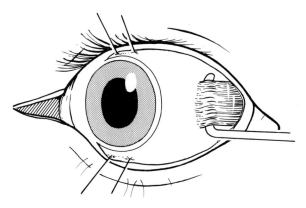

Fig. 4.5. Medial rectus isolated.

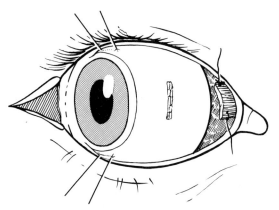

Fig. 4.6. Medial rectus detached, superior and inferior recti with bridle sutures.

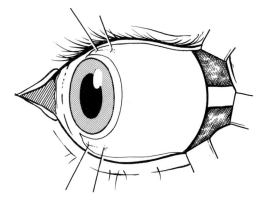

Fig. 4.7. The intraconal space exposed with the optic nerve on view.

a. Make a large lateral canthotomy (Fig. 4.4) as far as the orbital rim, cutting the lids full thickness after clamping with straight artery forceps.

b. Perform a peritomy for 270°, leaving the lateral 90° intact. Place a horizontal relieving incision in the conjunctiva medially as far as the plica semilunaris (Fig. 4.4).

c. Isolate the superior and inferior recti, and sling their tendons with heavy silk ties (Fig. 4.5).

d. Isolate the medial rectus (Fig. 4.5), tag its borders with 6/0 or 7/0 long-lasting absorbable sutures held with a bulldog clip, and detach its tendon from the sclera (Fig. 4.6).

e. Place retractors between the globe and the medial rectus to gain access to the intraconal space (Fig. 4.7). Traction on the inferior and superior rectus tie sutures will aid the exposure. Removal of

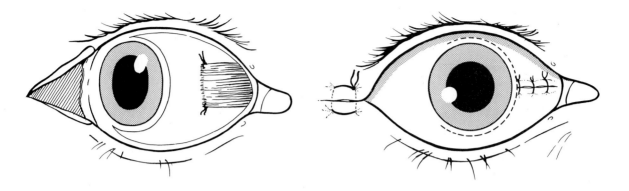

Fig. 4.8. Medial rectus reattached to the sclera.   **Fig. 4.9.** Conjunctiva and lateral canthotomy sutured.

the lid speculum may also allow the globe partially or completely to subluxate outside the lids, helping exposure.

 f. After obtaining a biopsy, removing the lesion or fenestrating the optic nerve sheath, reattach the medial rectus with the preplaced sutures (Fig. 4.8), close the conjunctiva with 6/0 catgut, and suture the canthotomy with horizontal mattress sutures of 6/0 silk (Fig. 4.9).

Complications

1. Transient diplopia is common due to underaction of the medial rectus, but vision usually recovers.

2. Pupil distortion may occur due to disruption of a long posterior ciliary nerve.

EXTRAPERIOSTEAL ANTERIOR ORBITOTOMY

Principle

An approach to a lesion is made via the extraperiosteal space without the removal of bone. This approach is also important in the management of orbital fractures.

Indications

1. Any lesion which has arisen from bone or invaded bone, or is confined to the extraperiosteal space (e.g. cholesterol granuloma, eosinophilic granuloma, sphenoid meningioma, extraperiosteal abscess or haematoma).

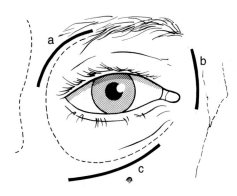

Fig. 4.10. Incisions for anterior extraperiosteal orbitotomy. a = brow incision; b = medial incision; c = inferior rim incision.

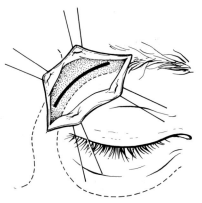

Fig. 4.11. Superior extraperiosteal anterior orbitotomy. Incision in periosteum marked.

2. Lesions that are confined to the orbit (i.e. not involving bone) should NOT be approached via the extraperiosteal space for incisional biopsy if malignancy is a possibility. This would open a surgical plane to tumour, and jeopardize safe removal later via exenteration if required.

Method

The method is the same for an approach along any of the orbital walls (Fig. 4.10), provided that normal structures such as supraorbital vessels and nerves and the lacrimal sac are identified and protected.

1. Make an incision along the orbital rim down to periosteum, and place traction sutures in the wound edges (Fig. 4.11).

2. Incise the periosteum several millimetres outside the orbital rim (Fig. 4.12a), and elevate it outwards for a few millimetres to facilitate later closure.

3. Elevate the periosteum towards the orbit, taking care as the rim is approached not to breach the periosteum. As the periosteum on the orbital walls is reached, it is elevated much more easily (Fig. 4.12b). Malleable retractors are useful to give access to the space created (Fig. 4.12c).

4. Having biopsied, drained or excised the lesion, place a drain (e.g. soft rubber glove drain) into the space and suture it to the wound edge as for trans-septal orbitotomy.

5. Close the periosteum with 4/0 long-lasting absorbable interrupted sutures (Fig. 4.13a).

6. The muscle is approximated with 5/0 chromic catgut, and the skin

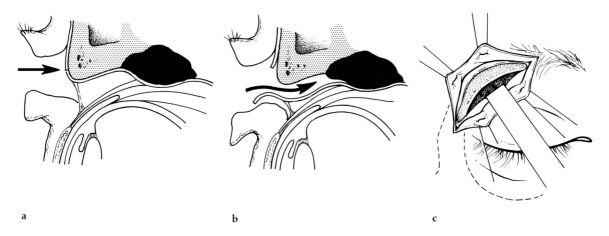

Fig. 4.12 a. Point of incision in periosteum. **b.** Periosteum elevated and extraperiosteal mass exposed. **c.** Periosteum elevated and retracted.

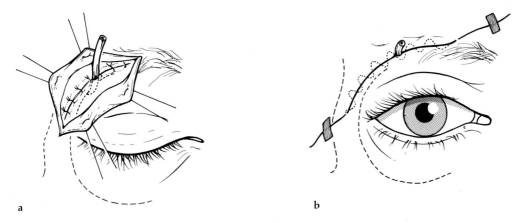

Fig. 4.13 a. Periosteum closed and drain tube inserted into extraperiosteal space. **b.** The wound closed and drain tube exiting the wound.

with 5/0 or 6/0 subcuticular nylon (Fig. 4.13b). The drain is removed at 24–48 hours (or longer if an abscess was present), depending on the amount of drainage, and the subcuticular suture tightened.

Further reading

Rootman, J., Stewart, B. and Goldberg, R. A. (1995). *Orbital Surgery. A Conceptual Approach.* Lippincott-Raven.

Rootman, J. (1988). Orbital surgery. In *Diseases of the Orbit* pp. 579–590. J B Lippincott.

Wright, J. E. (1985). Orbitotomy. In *Atlas of Ophthalmic Surgery* (P. Heilman and D. Paton, eds), pp. 12–18. Georg Thieme Verlag.

5

Lateral orbitotomy

Lateral orbitotomy is requird for a minority of orbital lesions. It is the standard approach to intraconal lesions (middle and posterior thirds of the orbit) and to benign lacrimal gland lesions. Krönlein in 1888 described removal of the lateral orbital wall to facilitate excision of a dermoid involving both the orbit and temporal fossa, and his name is most often associated with the operation.

Lateral orbitotomy

Principle
The lateral wall of the orbit is removed to facilitate access to an orbital lesion.

Indications

1. Intraconal lesions for complete removal (e.g. cavernous haemangioma) or incisional biopsy.
2. Pleomorphic adenomas of the lacrimal gland.
3. Other orbital lesions where an anterior approach would give inadequate access.
4. For large medially placed lesions, a lateral orbitotomy can be combined with an anterior medial orbitotomy for improved access.

Method

1. Exposure
   a. Mark the incision line (Fig. 5.1), beginning over the midpoint of the superior orbital rim (this may be above, below or within the eyebrow) and extending in a shallow sigmoid curve to a point above the zygomatic arch. An alternative is to use the lateral half of the upper lid crease and extend this across to join the usual incision line. This allows part of the scar to be hidden and also makes it easier to extend the exposure more medially to help with lesions in the superior orbit.

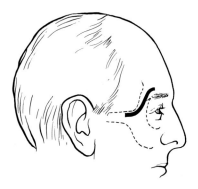

Fig. 5.1. Lateral orbitotomy incision.

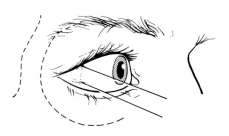

Fig. 5.2. Bridle suture under the lateral rectus.

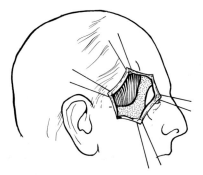

Fig. 5.3. Lateral orbital rim and zygomatic arch exposed.

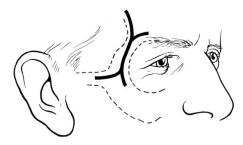

Fig. 5.4. Incisions in periosteum marked.

b. Place a transconjunctival 4/0 silk traction stitch under the lateral rectus tendon (Fig. 5.2).

c. Make an incision down to the level of the periosteum over the orbital rim, and raise the skin/muscle flaps in this plane over the temporalis fascia, zygomatic arch and towards the orbit so that the bony rim and arch are easily palpable. Place 3/0 silk traction sutures in the flaps to aid exposure (Fig. 5.3).

d. Incise the periosteum over the orbital rim, and extend this for 2–3 cm along the body of the zygoma towards the arch. Make relieving incisions in the periosteum above the superior temporal crest and along the inferolateral orbital rim (Fig. 5.4).

e. Elevate the periosteum over the bone to expose the whole of the orbital rim and superior edge of the zygomatic arch. Separate the anterior portion of the temporalis muscle from the back of the lateral orbital rim and retract it posteriorly out of its fossa to expose the outer aspect of the anterior part of the lateral orbital wall (Fig. 5.5).

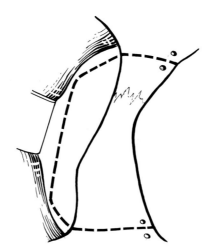

Fig. 5.5. Bone cuts and drill holes marked. Temporalis muscle retracted.

f. Elevate the periorbita on the internal aspect of the lateral orbital wall, the lacrimal fossa and superolateral orbit back as far as the inferior orbital fissure below.

g. Using an oscillating or reciprocating saw, make bone cuts superiorly and inferiorly through the thick orbital rim after preplacing drill holes above and below the cuts for later closure (Fig. 5.5). The upper bone cut should be above the zygomatico-frontal suture and in line with the superior orbital rim, slanting inferiorly into the temporal fossa to avoid entering the anterior cranial fossa. The lower cut is parallel to the upper border of the zygomatic arch.

h. Out-fracture the lateral orbital wall with bone holding forceps. If this is impossible, make a vertical bone cut in the thin bone of the lateral orbital wall behind the rim. Separate any remaining fibres of temporalis from the bone and place the free bone in saline.

i. Nibble the remaining thin bone of the lateral orbital wall back until the lateral orbital wall expands into the thicker greater wing of the sphenoid (Fig. 5.6a), exposing the periorbita of the lateral orbit (Fig. 5.6b).

j. Incise the periorbita circumferentially just behind the point where the rim was for the full extent of the exposure. Make a horizontal incision in the periorbita just below the lower pole of the lacrimal gland, making a T-shaped opening (Fig. 5.7). Dissect the flaps of periorbita from the underlying fat and lacrimal gland.

k. Locate the belly of the lateral rectus muscle just below the lower pole of the lacrimal gland, using traction on its bridle suture to

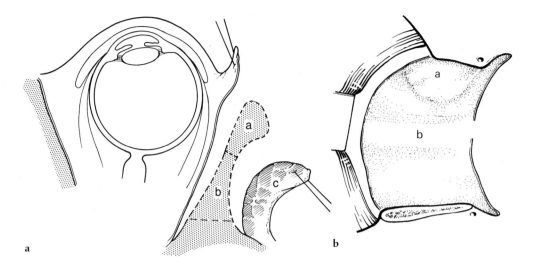

Fig. 5.6 a. Axial section of lateral orbitotomy. a = lateral orbital rim removed; b = lateral orbital wall nibbled back; c = temporalis muscle retracted.
b. Periorbita exposed after bone removed. a = lower pole of orbital lobe of lacrimal gland; b = position of lateral rectus muscle.

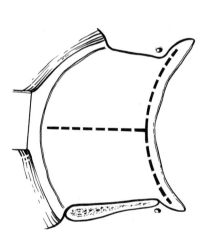

Fig. 5.7. Incisions in periorbita marked.

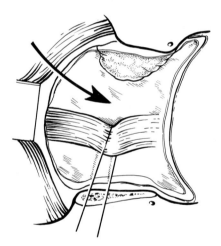

Fig. 5.8. Periorbita opened and retracted, lateral rectus retracted. Arrow marks point of entry into intraconal space.

aid in its location. Isolate the belly of the muscle and place a traction suture or tape around it (Fig. 5.8).

2. Intraorbital dissection (Principles. See also Chapter 4)

   a. Passing above or below the lateral rectus, enter the intraconal space by blunt dissection.

   b. Palpate the orbit with a finger to locate the tumour, the optic nerve and back of the globe.

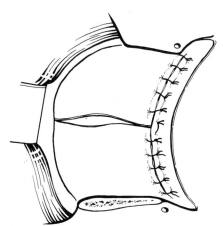

Fig. 5.9. Periorbita sutured anteriorly only.

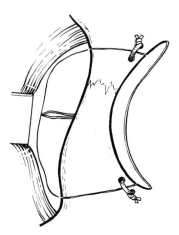

Fig. 5.10. The orbital rim replaced.

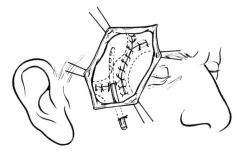

Fig. 5.11. The periosteal incisions closed and a drain tube in the temporal fossa, exiting through the skin.

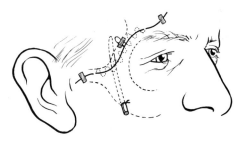

Fig. 5.12. Final wound closure.

    c. With careful blunt dissection, expose the lesion and separate it from the normal structures within the orbit.

    d. Obtain haemostasis with fine bipolar cautery, avoiding damage to important structures.

3. Closure

    a. Suture the anterior circumferential incision in the periorbita with interrupted 4/0 chromic catgut. Leave the horizontal incision open to allow any blood to escape into the temporal fossa (Fig. 5.9).

    b. Replace the bone after cleaning it of any fibrous tissue or muscle. Fine wire or heavy nylon (3/0) is passed through the drill holes and firmly tied (Fig. 5.10).

    c. Suture the periosteum on the outer aspect of the orbital rim with 3/0 chromic catgut or longer acting absorbable sutures (Fig. 5.11).

    d. Before closing the periosteum over the zygoma, place a suction drain into the temporal fossa to emerge below the incision line on the cheek (Fig. 5.11). Suture the drain to the skin.

e. Close the wound in two layers, using 4/0 chromic catgut to the deeper layers and 4/0 subcuticular nylon to the skin (Fig. 5.12).

f. Place a firm dressing over the wound, leaving the eye exposed so the vision may be monitored postoperatively.

g. The drain is removed at 24–48 hours, depending on the amount of blood draining.

Complications

1. *Infection.* This is extremely rare and should never occur. Parenteral antibiotics are given intraoperatively at the start of the procedure to reduce this risk. Antibiotics are not usually needed postoperatively.

2. *Haemorrhage.* Intraoperative haemorrhage may be avoided by the measures outlined in Chapter 4, by careful dissection, and by bipolar cautery to nonvital structures before they are cut. If it does occur, careful bipolar cautery or pressure is used. Postoperative haemorrhage is usually minor, and is managed by the suction drain. If a significant haemorrhage occurs there will be pain, increased proptosis, ophthalmoplegia and possibly reduced vision. If vision is threatened the wound may need to be reopened and clot evacuated. This is rare.

3. *Damage to orbital structures.* Almost any structure within the orbit may be damaged during surgery, but the following occur most frequently:

    a. *Lateral rectus palsy.* This is common, usually mild and recovers in most cases. Squint surgery is rarely required.

    b. *Pupillary distortion.* This occurs from damage to the posterior ciliary nerves or ciliary ganglion. It may recover, or a tonic pupil may result.

    c. *Blindness.* This is uncommon, and occurs most frequently with posterior lesions, those attached to the optic nerve, and where damage occurs to the ophthalmic artery or central retinal artery. Central retinal artery occlusion may occur with raised intraorbital pressure from haemorrhage and/or oedema. If no clot can be removed, high dose steroids may help relieve pressure from oedema. Choroidal infarction can occur from posterior ciliary artery damage and compromise vision.

    d. *Ptosis and diplopia.* Any extraocular muscle or its nerve may be damaged. A full 6 months is allowed to elapse before offering corrective surgery for any symptomatic residual deficit that shows no signs of recovery. Ptosis may occur from damage to the aponeurosis or its lateral horn.

Other surgical approaches to the orbit

Detailed description of these procedures is beyond the scope of this book.

TRANSCRANIAL

For lesions at the orbital apex or extending intracranially, transcranial surgery may be required. This is performed in conjunction with a neurosurgeon.

EXTENDED ANTEROLATERAL AND SUPERIOR ORBITOTOMY

The amount of bone removed to gain access to the orbit may be increased by removing the superior orbital rim in combination with the lateral orbital wall, or by removal of the superior orbital rim and orbital roof via a transfrontal craniotomy. A neurosurgeon is again required.

Further reading

McNab, A. A. and Wright, J. E. (1990). Lateral orbitotomy – a review. *Aust. N. Z. J. Ophthalmol.*, **18**, 281–286.

Rootman, J., Stewart, B. and Goldberg, R. A. (1995). *Orbital Surgery. A Conceptual Approach.* Lippincott-Raven.

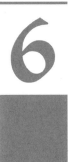

Orbital exenteration

Exenteration of the orbit is a disfiguring procedure, and its usual indication is in the management of malignant disease. Patients therefore need careful and sympathetic counselling before embarking on such surgery. They should be aware of the radical differences between exenteration and enucleation or evisceration of the globe, as many patients will assume that they will wear an artificial eye similar to those most often seen in the community. The nature and quality of the prostheses available should be explained. In addition, there will often be loss of sensation throughout the first division of the trigeminal nerve.

The choice of type of exenteration will depend on the nature and position of the lesion that necessitates the procedure. Under no circumstances should the effectiveness and completeness of the excision be compromised in order to simplify the surgery or the reconstruction. If the lids or periosteum need to be excised for purposes of adequate excision, then this should be done.

Exenteration of the orbit, including the lids

Principle
The eyelids and the whole of the orbital contents are removed, including the periorbita.

Indications

1. Orbital malignancy

   a. Primary orbital malignancies.

   b. Secondary orbital malignancies arising from the lids, conjunctiva or globe, and involving the orbit secondarily (e.g. basal cell carcinoma of the lids invading the orbit). Malignancies invading the orbit from adjacent structures (such as the paranasal sinuses) will require orbital exenteration in combination with radical craniofacial surgery, if feasible. This is beyond the scope of this text.

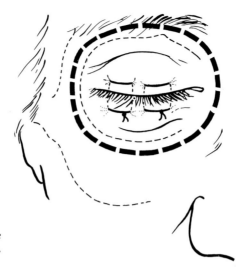

Fig. 6.1. Exenteration including the eyelids. Incision over the orbital rim, lids sutured.

2. Orbital infection. Fungal infection (usually mucormycosis). This will usually require concomitant radical sinus surgery, and sometimes even wider excision of infected and devitalized tissue.

3. Pain relief. Occasionally, non-malignant disease processes of the orbit, such as idiopathic orbital inflammation (pseudotumour), may cause unremitting pain that is difficult to control. Exenteration of the orbit may be used as a last resort in such instances.

Method

1. Suture the lids together with some 3/0 or 4/0 nylon or silk.

2. Make a skin incision along the whole circumference of the orbital margin, passing medial to the medial canthus, and well outside any previous incisions used to obtain biopsy material from a malignancy (Fig. 6.1).

3. Deepen the incision to the periosteum. Cutting diathermy simplifies this and reduces blood loss.

4. Incise (or cut with diathermy) the periosteum over the orbital rim.

5. Elevate the periosteum over the orbital rim and into the orbit. Diathermy and divide all neurovascular bundles passing through foramina of the orbit, and divide the nasolacrimal duct as it enters its bony canal (Fig. 6.2).

6. Continue the periosteal elevation to the orbital apex and superior and inferior orbital fissures. Tissue passing through the inferior orbital fissure can be divided using cautery.

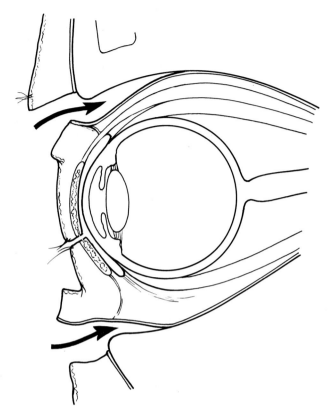

Fig. 6.2. The periosteum incised over the rims and the extraperiosteal space entered.

7. When only the structures passing through the superior orbital fissure and optic foramen remain, divide the orbital contents as far posterior as possible (Fig. 6.3), using stout curved scissors, a curved-tipped cutting diathermy needle or a very strong wire snare. Be careful not to puncture the delicate medial orbital wall. If significant tissue remains at the orbital apex (which is usual when scissors are used) this can then be removed separately.

8. Obtain haemostasis; use bipolar cautery in preference to monopolar cautery as the cavernous sinus and middle cranial fossa are only a few millimetres away.

9. Place tulle gras on the bare bone, fill the socket with absorbent gauze and apply a firm pressure dressing for 3–4 days. Change this dressing and clean the socket with dilute hypochlorite (Eusol) solution once or twice daily. When granulations appear from the fissures and margins and begin to cover the bone, this can be reduced in frequency. The socket generally epithelializes in 6–8 weeks.

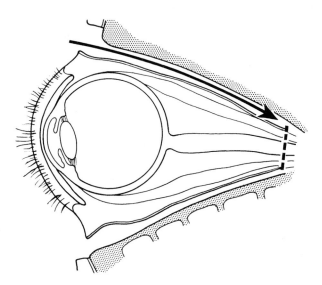

Fig. 6.3. The contents of the orbit transected as far posteriorly as possible.

10. An alternative is to line the socket with split skin grafts. This gives more rapid healing, but the skin often desquamates excessive keratin, which can be malodorous and requires frequent cleaning. The transfer of a flap of temporalis muscle through a hole in the lateral orbital wall can be used to fill some of the socket, and then covered with split skin. However, a shallow socket is no advantage when a prosthesis is fitted, and the hollow temporal fossa may be a cosmetic problem.

11. Have the patient fitted with a spectacle-mounted prosthesis when healing is complete. If available, titanium pegs fixed to the orbital rim can be used to mount the prosthesis, but the lifeless appearance is more obvious when the prosthesis is not hidden behind spectacles.

Complications

1. *Cerebrospinal fluid leak.* This is uncommon. A flap of temporalis muscle can be brought through the lateral orbital wall and sutured to the orbital rim. Other flaps such as a midline forehead flap can also be used. Systemic antibiotics should be given.

2. *Fistula into the paranasal sinuses.* This may cause problems with mucus accumulation behind the prosthesis. Once the socket has epithelialized, a flap of skin can be rotated over the defect and the donor site allowed to granulate. Larger flaps (temporalis or forehead) may occasionally be needed.

Exenteration sparing the lids

Principle

The contents of the orbit are removed, sparing some or all of the skin of the eyelids.

Indications

1. Primary orbital malignancy confined to the orbit, without involvement of the eyelids, provided that sparing the lids does not reduce the chances of the procedure being curative.

2. Secondary orbital malignancy which has spread from the globe or conjunctiva, but does not involve the eyelids.

Method

1. Suture the lid margins together.

2. Make an incision a few millimetres outside the lid margins, extending in a horizontal line beyond the orbital margin medially and laterally (Fig. 6.4).

3. In the lids, deepen the incision to beneath the orbicularis muscle, then dissect in this plane towards the orbital margins so that a flap of skin and orbicularis is preserved. If one lid only is preserved, the other is excised as for exenteration including the eyelids (Fig. 6.5).

4. Retract the flaps to expose the orbital rim, and incise the periosteum

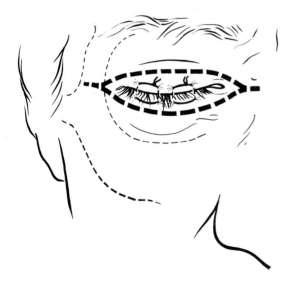

Fig. 6.4. Exenteration sparing the eyelid skin. Incision marked.

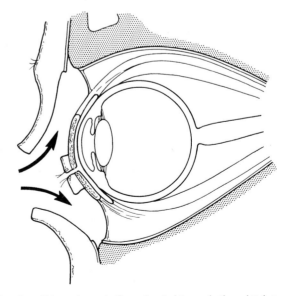

Fig. 6.5. Skin and muscle flaps elevated towards the orbital rim.

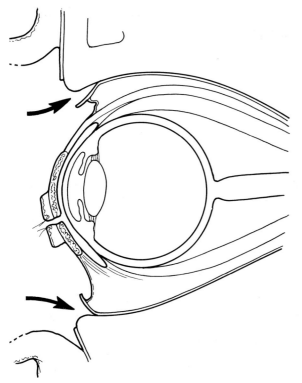

Fig. 6.6. The periosteum incised and elevated.

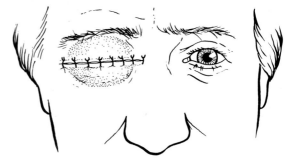

Fig. 6.7. The residual lid skin and orbicularis sutured together.

over the orbital rim (Fig. 6.6). Proceed as for exenteration with excision of the eyelids (steps 5 to 8).

5. If both lids have been preserved, suture them together without tension in two layers using a long-acting absorbable suture for the muscle and 5/0 silk or nylon for the skin (Fig. 6.7). (If only one lid has been preserved, close the defect as far as possible without tension, drape the skin over the bone and hold it in place for several days with a firm dressing. Allow the remainder to granulate.)

6. Apply a firm dressing that does not place too much tension on the wound.

7. An alternative is to intentionally place a hole in the floor of the orbit into the maxillary antrum before closing the wound. This provides drainage, and with respiration the skin and muscle flaps are drawn back into the socket.

Complications

1. *Wound breakdown.* Allow the defect to granulate and heal by secondary intention.

2. *Haematoma behind the flaps.* This is common, and can either be allowed spontaneously to resorb or aspirated with a large bore needle.

Anterior exenteration

Principle
The anterior contents of the orbit (globe and posterior lamellae of lids and the entire conjunctival sac) are excised. This differs from exenteration of the orbit with sparing of the lids in that the periorbita and the posterior orbital contents are preserved. A shallow skin-lined socket results.

Indications
This procedure is primarily indicated for conjunctival malignancy not manageable by local measures, or for sebaceous carcinoma with extensive intraepithelial (pagetoid) spread.

Method

1. Suture the lid margins together.

2. Make an incision several millimetres outside the lid margin and extend it horizontally across the medial and lateral orbital margins. (Fig. 6.4).

3. Deepen the incision to beneath the orbicularis muscle and dissect in this plane towards the orbital rims. (Fig. 6.5).

4. At the orbital margins, continue the dissection into the orbit by opening the orbital septum near its junction with the orbital margins (Fig. 6.8).

5. Isolate the levator palpebrae superioris beneath the pre-aponeurotic fat pad, and divide it behind Whitnall's ligament. Beneath it lies the superior rectus. This also should be divided, but well back from the superior fornix to avoid opening the conjunctival sac. The superior oblique tendon will be found in the superomedial quadrant, and is now divided.

6. In the inferomedial orbit, locate the inferior oblique as it enters the medial border of the capsulopalpebral head of the inferior rectus and divide it. The inferior rectus is then located and divided.

7. The medial and lateral rectus muscle are similarly found and divided.

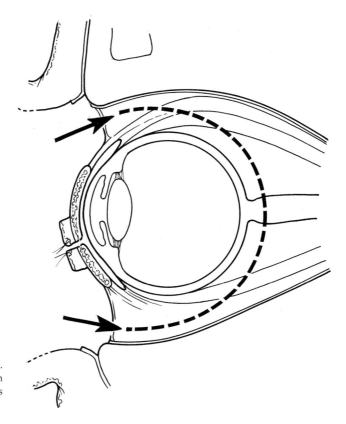

Fig. 6.8. Anterior partial exenteration. The incision in the orbital septum made, and the anterior orbital contents removed.

8. The medial and lateral palpebral ligaments are divided.

9. The lacrimal gland should be included in the excision by elevating it out of its fossa. Similarly, the lacrimal sac is removed as part of the block excision and the nasolacrimal duct is divided as it enters its bony canal.

10. The frontal nerve and its anterior branches (supraorbital and supratrochlear) may be preserved and protected during the excision by a malleable retractor. This preserves sensation to the forehead and scalp.

11. Using heavy curved scissors, divide the optic nerve along with any fascial and neurovascular attachments just behind the globe. If any extraocular muscles have not yet been found, they can be divided at this point.

12. Close the orbicularis with long-acting absorbable 5/0 sutures, and the skin with 5/0 silk or nylon (Fig. 6.7).

Complications

These are similar to exenteration of the orbit with sparing of the lids.

Exenteration with removal of orbital bone

Principle
The orbital contents are excised along with a portion of the orbital rim or walls

Indications
Removal of bone in combination with the soft tissues of the orbit is indicated for tumours that are fixed to the bone. These may be seen in advanced eyelid tumours invading the orbit, possibly in some lacrimal gland carcinomas, or in tumours arising from adjacent structures such as the paranasal sinuses and secondarily involving the orbit. Description of these latter two groups is beyond the scope of this text.

Complications

These are similar to those for other types of exenteration but additional potential complications will depend on the area of bone excised.

Method

1. Carefully assess the area to be excised on the basis of clinical findings and imaging by CT or MRI.
2. Mark the skin to be excised and incise down to bone.
3. Mobilize the contents of the orbit in a subperiosteal plane as described above, except over the area where bone is also to be removed. Soft tissues (and tumour) are left attached to the bone at this point and for an adequate margin around the area.
4. Bone cuts are made through the orbital rim and walls, and the orbital contents and attached bone removed *en bloc*.
5. Details of each operation will vary depending on the type and position of the tumour, but appropriate assistance should be obtained from other specialists as needed.
6. Reconstruction will depend on the area excised, but may include skin grafts or local flaps such as a midline forehead flap, temporalis flap or vascularized free flap.

7

Orbital decompression

Orbital decompression is most commonly indicated for severe thyroid eye disease with optic neuropathy. There are several ways of decompressing the orbit, each with advantages and disadvantages. The comparative merits of these will not be discussed in detail, and only those techniques that an ophthalmologist may be expected to perform will be discussed. Transcranial decompression is rarely performed now, and has no distinct advantage over other methods. The transantral approach to the floor and medial wall is a useful technique, which can be performed in conjunction with an ENT surgeon. Another approach that has been introduced recently is to perform an orbital decompression using endoscopic transnasal techniques. Again, this allows only decompression of the floor and medial wall, and requires special experience in this type of surgery, the assistance of ENT colleagues and additional instrumentation.

For optic nerve compression, the most important aspect of the decompression is the medial wall in its most posterior part, where compression is maximal.

Principle
One, two or three orbital walls are decompressed, to relieve pressure on the optic nerve and reduce proptosis.

Indications
1. Thyroid eye disease with optic neuropathy, or with sight-threatening corneal exposure not treatable by simpler methods.
2. Optic nerve compression due to inoperable neoplastic or inflammatory tumours of the orbit, where an attempt to conserve vision is desired.
3. Cosmetically disfiguring proptosis, usually associated with severe thyroid eye disease.

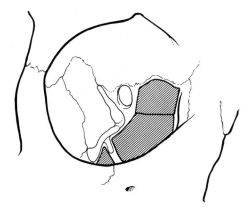

Fig. 7.1. Orbital decompression, floor and medial wall. The bone to be removed marked.

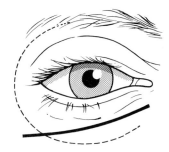

Fig. 7.2. Skin incision for floor and medial wall decompression.

Methods

1. Medial wall and floor (Fig. 7.1) via:

    a. Transcutaneous lower lid incision

    b. Transconjunctival approach

    c. Separate medial and inferior skin incisions

    d. Transantral or endoscopic techniques (not discussed)

2. Combinations of medial wall, floor and lateral wall via:

    a. Transconjunctival approach

    b. Separate medial and lateral skin incisions

    c. Coronal approach.

Transcutaneous lower lid approach to floor and medial wall decompression

The floor and medial orbital wall can be quickly and easily reached through a single lower lid incision.

Method

1. Make a sloping incision in the lower lid, starting near the medial canthus and extending down over the inferior orbital rim (Fig. 7.2).

2. Divide orbicularis, and expose the periosteum over the inferior orbital rim for the full extent of the rim (Fig. 7.3).

3. Divide the periosteum just outside the orbit (Fig. 7.3), elevate a small frill inferiorly and then raise the periosteum over the orbital rim and

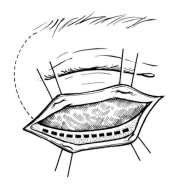

Fig. 7.3. The orbital rim exposed and the periosteal incision marked.

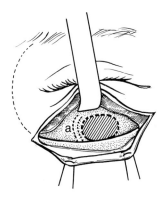

Fig. 7.4. The periorbita elevated to expose the orbital floor, and the commencement of the removal of bone medial to the infraorbital nerve (a).

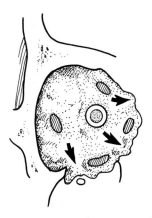

Fig. 7.5. Coronal section with the floor and medial wall removed, and the orbital contents prolapsing into the space created.

into the floor of the orbit. Be careful not to damage the periorbita and allow fat to prolapse, as it will obscure the view and make the surgery more difficult.

4. Elevate the periorbita up the medial wall of the orbit behind the posterior lacrimal crest and as far posterior as possible.

5. Locate the infraorbital neurovascular bundle and fracture the floor medial to it (Fig. 7.4). Remove the thin bone of the floor piecemeal as far as the posterior wall of the maxillary antrum and up to the infraorbital canal. Carefully deroof the canal and remove any bone lateral to the canal so that the nerve and vessels are suspended across the roof of the antrum.

6. Infracture the thin medial wall and remove it and the lining of the ethmoid air cells. A useful landmark is the posterior wall of the antrum. The medial wall extends for another 1 cm or so posteriorly.

7. Carefully incise the periorbita anteroposteriorly, medially and inferiorly to allow free prolapse of orbital fat into the space created (Fig. 7.5).

8. Close the periosteum over the inferior rim with 4/0 chromic catgut or similar suture.

9. Close the wound in two layers using 5/0 chromic catgut for the muscle and 6/0 nylon subcuticular for the skin (Fig. 7.6).

Advantages

1. A simple and quick approach to the floor and medial wall.

2. Less conjunctival oedema postoperatively.

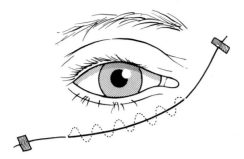

Fig. 7.6. The skin closure.

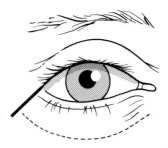

Fig. 7.7. Orbital decompression of floor and medial wall via the inferior fornix. Lateral canthotomy and inferior fornix incision.

Disadvantages

1. Difficult exposure of the superior and posterior parts of the medial orbital wall and the ethmoidal vessels.

2. Possibly increased incidence of worsening ocular motility compared to medial and lateral wall decompression, or three wall decompression.

3. Visible scar if performed for purely cosmetic reasons.

Transconjunctival decompression of floor and medial wall

The orbital floor is easily accessed via the inferior conjunctival fornix. The medial wall may also be exposed via the inferior fornix, or a separate cutaneous incision may be made to give greater exposure of the medial wall. A further technique allows the medial wall to be exposed via a medial conjunctival incision (see below).

Method

1. Make a sloping, full-thickness lateral canthotomy and release the inferior limb of the lateral canthal tendon (Fig. 7.7).

2. Incise the conjunctiva in the inferior fornix directly down to the orbital floor just behind the rim, placing a large retractor against the globe into the fornix and pressing onto the floor to aid exposure (Fig. 7.8). Alternatively, dissect bluntly with scissors in a plane anterior to the conjunctiva and lower eyelid retractors, then divide these several millimetres below the inferior border of the tarsal plate as far as the lacrimal punctum. Then dissect in the plane between orbital septum and orbicularis down to the inferior orbital rim.

3. Incise the periorbita on the inferior orbital rim. Patients with severe

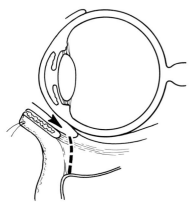

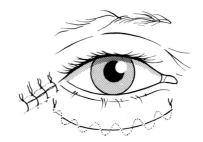

Fig. 7.8. Incision down to the orbital rim through fornix.

Fig. 7.9. Wound closure.

thyroid eye disease often have increased amounts of extraorbital fat overlying the orbital rim that also needs to be incised. Elevate the periosteum into the floor and up the medial wall as above.

4. Proceed as for a transcutaneous approach.
5. Close the fornix with interrupted or continuous 6/0 plain catgut sutures, and the lateral canthotomy with interrupted sutures in two layers, recreating the canthal angle carefully (Fig. 7.9).

Advantage
This gives a small cutaneous incision.

Disadvantages

1. Poor exposure of the medial wall and ethmoidal vessels.
2. Prolapsing orbital fat from the earliest stage of the operation as the orbital septum is usually opened with the fornix incision.
3. Difficult access to the inferior fornix if proptosis severe.
4. More conjunctival oedema postoperatively.

Transconjunctival medial orbital decompression

The medial orbital wall may be accessed via a conjunctival incision between the caruncle and plica. The distance to the medial wall from here is small, and the dissection avoids detaching structures from the posterior lacrimal crest and also leaves the lacrimal system undisturbed.

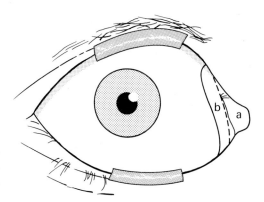

Fig. 7.10. The conjunctival incision for a medial transconjunctival decompression (dotted line). a = caruncle; b = plica semilunaris.

Method

1. Place an eyelid speculum to widely separate the lids.

2. Make a conjunctival incision between the caruncle and the plica semilunaris, extending it as far superiorly and inferiorly as possible (Fig. 7.10). If an inferior conjunctival fornix incision is present, the two incisions may be joined.

3. Bluntly dissect towards a point behind the posterior lacrimal crest, spreading with scissors until the periosteum is reached. A probe in a lacrimal canaliculus and into the lacrimal sac may aid in determining the direction to proceed with the dissection.

4. Place malleable retractors to expose the periosteum of the medial wall behind the posterior lacrimal crest, incise it vertically, then elevate the periosteum posteriorly to expose the medial orbital wall and ethmoidal vessels.

5. If the inferior fornix has been used to access the orbital floor, the incisions may be joined to expose widely the floor and medial walls. The periosteal incisions must be joined by detaching the inferior oblique muscle from its origin lateral to the lacrimal sac, and then extending the periosteal incision up behind the lacrimal sac to join the medial periosteal incision.

6. Proceed to decompress the medial wall as described above.

7. Close the conjunctival incision with several interrupted 6/0 plain catgut sutures.

Advantages

1. Avoidance of a cutaneous scar.

2. No disruption to the lacrimal system or attachments of the medial canthal structures to the posterior lacrimal crest.

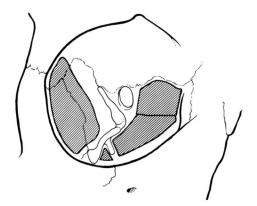

Fig. 7.11. The bone removed in a three wall orbital decompression.

Disadvantages

1. Less wide exposure of the medial wall than a transcutaneous approach.

2. More conjunctival and caruncular oedema postoperatively, which may be prolonged.

Transconjunctival three wall orbital decompression

The lateral wall may be decompressed via a transconjunctival approach with a canthotomy incision as well as decompressing the floor and medial wall by either of the techniques outlined above (Fig. 7.11), or the lateral and medial walls may be decompressed leaving the floor intact.

Method

1. Make a sloping lateral canthotomy incision as in Fig. 7.7, but make it a little longer until it extends well over the lateral orbital rim.

2. Open the inferior fornix (as above) and incise the periosteum over the inferior orbital rim as far as the canthotomy incision.

3. Expose the periosteum over the lateral orbital rim by dissecting in a plane superficial to it, extending superiorly over the orbital rim as far as possible and posteriorly over the anterior part of the temporalis fascia and zygomatic arch.

4. Extend the periosteal incision from the inferior orbital rim around to the lateral orbital rim, and add a relieving incision laterally over the zygomatic arch. To extend the exposure superiorly over the lateral orbital rim, it helps to proceed piece by piece, incising some periosteum and then elevating it and repeating this step until sufficient lateral orbital rim is exposed.

5. Elevate the periosteum to expose the lateral orbital rim and detach the temporalis fascia from the posterior edge of the rim. Cutting diathermy aids in this.

6. Elevate the periosteum into the orbit to expose the medial aspect of the lateral orbital wall.

7. Make two bone cuts with a bone saw as for a lateral orbitotomy. The superior bone cut may not be as high as with a standard lateral orbitotomy incision.

8. Outfracture the lateral orbital rim and remove it by cutting any temporalis muscle from its lateral part.

9. Remove the thinner bone of the lateral wall with bone nibblers, and then use a burr to remove bone of the thicker greater wing of the sphenoid. Bleeding from this cancellous bone is common, with large diploic channels present, and is best controlled with bone wax. Bone may be removed as far inferiorly as the inferior orbital fissure, and superiorly into the lacrimal gland fossa. Small areas of dura may be exposed. The bone of the lateral wall may be removed with a burr and bone nibblers without removing the lateral rim, but the exposure is more difficult.

10. Incise the periorbita laterally to allow free prolapse of orbital contents into the space created.

11. Decompress the floor and medial wall as described above. Thin the lateral rim to a strut and replace it using heavy sutures through small burr holes or mini-plates.

12. Close the periosteum over the lateral rim, being careful to position the lateral canthal structures correctly, then close the wounds as above.

Advantages

1. Avoidance of large cutaneous incisions.
2. Possibly lower risk of induced diplopia, particularly if the medial and lateral walls are decompressed, and the floor is either left intact or decompressed in its posterior half only.

Disadvantages

1. More difficult exposure of the lateral wall than by standard lateral orbitotomy.

2. Increased conjunctival oedema compared to transcutaneous techniques.

Separate medial and inferior skin incisions for floor and medial wall decompression

A separate medial skin incision provides the best exposure of the medial orbital wall, and is particularly indicated when optic neuropathy is present. It may be used in combination with any of the above approaches.

Method

1. Decompress the orbital floor as for transcutaneous approach.

2. Make a separate incision medially starting at the medial end of the eyebrow and running down the lateral side of the nose about midway between the canthus and the midline (Fig. 7.12).

3. Incise the periosteum and elevate it to expose the lacrimal fossa and the whole of the medial orbital wall (Fig. 7.13). Locate the anterior and posterior ethmoid vessels and nerves as they exit the orbit and diathermy them before cutting them. These mark the upper extent of the medial orbital wall.

4. Infracture the medial wall behind the posterior lacrimal crest, and remove the bony medial wall and ethmoid air cells piecemeal until in continuity with the decompression of the floor. The posterior extent of bone removal is marked by the thicker bone of the lateral wall of the sphenoid sinus, which lies 35–40 mm from the anterior lacrimal crest.

5. If the heavier strut of bone between the floor and medial wall is left intact, the risk of diplopia may be reduced. In addition, the drainage

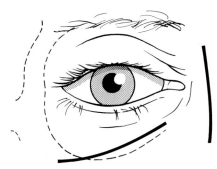

Fig. 7.12. Orbital decompression of floor and medial wall with separate incisions.

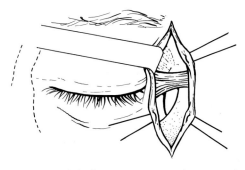

Fig. 7.13. Medical incision exposing the anterior limb of the medial canthal tendon.

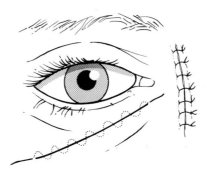

Fig. 7.14. Wound closure.

of the maxillary antrum is high up on its medial wall, and it may be obstructed by orbital fat if this strut is removed.

6. Incise the periorbita to allow free prolapse of orbital contents.

7. Close the wounds in layers (Fig. 7.14).

Advantages

1. Much better exposure of the medial wall and ethmoidal vessels, allowing a more thorough decompression of the orbital apex when optic neuropathy is present.

2. Less conjunctival oedema than with transconjunctival approaches.

Disadvantages

1. Two incisions required.

2. Visible scars.

Combined medial and lateral transcutaneous decompression

The medial and lateral orbital walls may be decompressed by separate cutaneous incisions (Fig. 7.15), using a standard lateral orbitotomy incision for the lateral wall rather than a lateral canthotomy as described above.

Method

1. Proceed as for lateral orbitotomy until the whole of the lateral orbital rim and thinner mid-portion of the wall is removed.

2. Using a burr, remove the thicker bone of the greater wing of the sphenoid until a thin layer of bone remains over the dura of the middle cranial fossa or a small piece of dura is exposed. This may

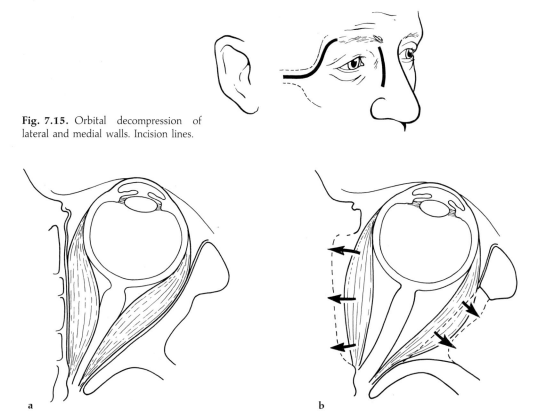

Fig. 7.15. Orbital decompression of lateral and medial walls. Incision lines.

a

b

Fig. 7.16 a. Axial section demonstrating optic nerve compression by enlarging muscles. **b.** Combined medial and lateral wall decompression.

extend inferiorly as far as the inferior orbital fissure and superiorly into the area of the lacrimal gland fossa.

3. Obtain haemostasis with cautery and bone wax – large diploic vessels in the bone are common.

4. A segment of temporalis muscle (preserving its overlying fascia) lateral to the decompression may be removed to provide more space for the prolapsing orbital contents.

5. Incise the periorbita anteroposteriorly in several places, and join these to allow free prolapse of orbital fat (Fig. 7.16).

7. Nibble the removed lateral wall until only a thin strut of bone remains.

8. Fix this strut in a position slightly lateral and anterior to its former position, to increase the decompressive effect (Fig. 7.17). Miniplates

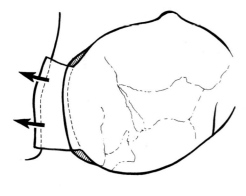

Fig. 7.17. The lateral orbital rim may be shifted laterally for more effect.

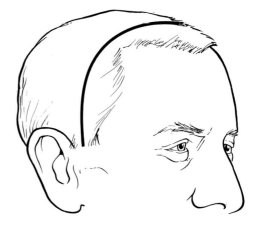

Fig. 7.18. Coronal incision for orbital decompression.

may aid this. Any contour deformity can be corrected with acrylic or bone cement, or similar material.

9. Do a medial decompression as above via a separate incision.

Advantages

1. Better exposure of the medial wall and ethmoidal vessels.
2. Possibly reduced ocular motility disturbance, compared to medial wall and floor decompressions.

Disadvantages

1. Two separate incisions and a longer operating time.
2. Visible scars.

Coronal approach to orbital decompression

A coronal approach gives good access to the medial and lateral walls via a remote and hidden incision.

Method

1. Make a coronal incision from ear to ear, beginning in front of the ear near to its attachment to the scalp (Fig. 7.18). Place haemostatic clips on the wound edges.
2. Raise the scalp down to the superior orbital rims and over the temporalis fascia and lateral orbital rims.

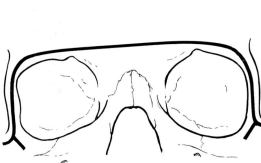

Fig. 7.19. Periosteal incisions.

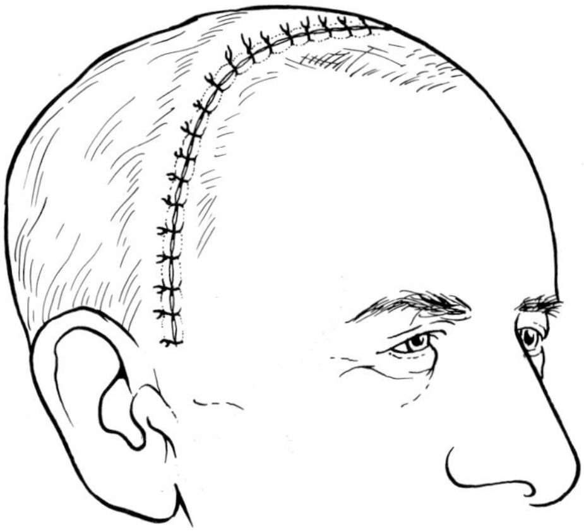

Fig. 7.20. Wound closure.

3. Expose the zygomatic arch by following the deeper layer of the temporalis fascia, thus avoiding the upper branches of the facial nerve.

4. Incise the periosteum above the orbital rim (Fig. 7.19), and elevate it towards the orbit. If the supraorbital neurovascular bundle is within a bony canal, use a small osteotome to free it from within its canal.

5. Expose the medial wall, the roof and lateral wall (as for lateral orbitotomy) and proceed to decompress the medial and lateral walls as above.

6. The floor can be reached via the side or by a separate inferior incision, if it is desired to decompress it as well.

7. Close the periosteum with 4/0 chromic gut interrupted sutures or longer acting absorbables, and the scalp in layers using staples for the skin if available (Fig. 7.20). A drain tube may be placed in the temporal fossa.

Advantages

1. Hidden scar (avoid this approach in balding men).
2. Good exposure of the medial wall and ethmoidal vessels.

Disadvantages

1. Difficult exposure of the floor without a separate incision.
2. Prolonged operating time.

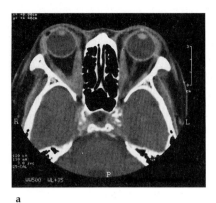
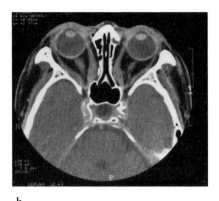

a   b

Fig. 7.21 a. Preoperative axial CT scan of a patient undergoing decompression of the medial wall and floor.
b. Postoperative axial CT scan showing displacement of the medial orbital contents into the space created by decompression of the medial wall. The patient had an esotropia postoperatively.

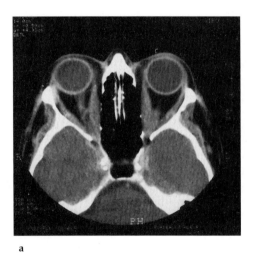
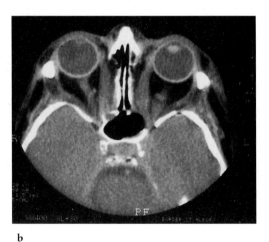

a   b

Fig. 7.22 a. Preoperative axial CT scan of a patient undergoing medial and lateral wall decompression.
b. Postoperative axial CT scan showing symmetrical displacement of the medial and lateral orbital contents into the spaces created by medial and lateral decompression (so-called 'balanced decompression'). There was no worsening of motility after surgery.

Complications of orbital decompression

1. *Failure to decompress the optic nerve and improve vision.* In this case, walls not already decompressed can be attacked, or alternative treatment with radiotherapy or immunosuppression can be given. If optic neuropathy is the indication for decompression, it is wise to increase corticosteroids over the perioperative period.

2. *Haemorrhage.* This usually occurs from ethmoidal or infraorbital

vessels. If it occurs intraoperatively, every attempt is made to stop it with bipolar diathermy. Postoperatively, bleeding occurs into the sinuses and rarely requires evacuation. A drain tube may be inserted if bleeding is difficult to control, and should be used routinely for lateral and coronal approaches. If vision is compromised post-operatively and haemorrhage is present, wounds should be opened, any clot evacuated, and drains placed.

3. *Numbness and paraesthesia.* This may occur in the distribution of any of the nerves exposed: supraorbital, infraorbital, ethmoidal and zygomatic. It usually diminishes in time or disappears.

4. *Infection.* Despite opening the contents of the orbit to the potentially infected paranasal sinuses, this complication is surprisingly rare. Removal of the strut between the floor and medial wall may allow fat to prolapse down and obstruct the meatus of the maxillary antrum.

5. *Diplopia.* New or worsening diplopia is the commonest complication of orbital decompression, and its frequency has been reported to be as high as 60%. The incidence appears to be higher when a medial wall and floor decompression is performed than when a medial and lateral decompression is chosen, with or without a limited floor decompression (a so-called 'balanced decompression' – compare Fig. 7.21a, b with Fig. 7.22a, b). Increased diplopia also occurs when ocular motility disturbances are present preoperatively, or when marked extraocular muscle enlargement is present.

6. *Chemosis.* Conjunctival oedema may increase after orbital decompression, especially when transconjunctival approaches are used. The oedema may be prolonged.

Further reading

Garrity, J. A., Fatourechi, V., Bergstralh, E. J. *et al.* (1993). Results of transantral orbital decompression in 428 patients with severe Graves' ophthalmopathy. *Am. J. Ophthalmol.,* **116**, 533–547.

Lyons, C. J. and Rootman, J. (1994). Orbital decompression for disfiguring exophthalmos in thyroid orbitopathy. *Ophthalmology,* **101**, 223–230.

McNab, A. (1997). Orbital decompression for thyroid orbitopathy. *Aust. N. Z. J. Ophthalmol*, **25**, 26–32.

Mourits, M., Koornneef, L., Wiersinga, W. M. *et al.* (1990). Orbital decompression for Graves' ophthalmopathy by inferomedial, by inferomedial plus lateral and by coronal approach. *Ophthalmology,* **97**, 636–641.

8

Orbital trauma

This chapter deals with fractures of the orbital floor and medial wall occurring in isolation from orbital rim and other facial fractures (blow-out fractures), orbital haemorrhage and traumatic optic neuropathy. It is recognized that orbital floor and medial wall fractures often occur as part of more complex facial fractures, but the management of these is beyond the scope of this book and demands the combined skills of plastic, neurosurgical, faciomaxillary and ophthalmic surgeons. However, pure blow-out fractures should be managed readily by the ophthalmologist, with or without the assistance of other specialists.

Orbital fractures

DIAGNOSIS

Orbital blow-out fractures are usually caused by blunt trauma to the orbital contents and rim from such objects as fists or balls of similar size (cricket, tennis, baseball, etc.).

Symptoms

1. Vertical diplopia in up or down gaze, in the primary position, or any combination of these.

2. Paraesthesia in the distribution of the infraorbital nerve.

3. Enophthalmos which may not be apparent until swelling and bruising has settled.

4. If the medial wall is also fractured or an isolated medial blow-out occurs (much less common), there may be restriction of horizontal movements.

5. Subcutaneous and orbital emphysema may occur after nose blowing, and the patient should be warned to avoid this.

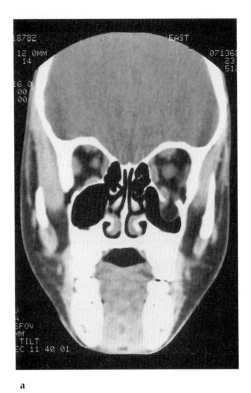

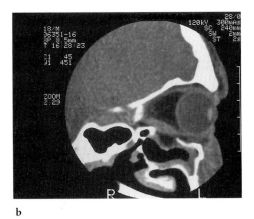

a   b

Fig. 8.1 a. Coronal CT scan of a blow-out fracture of the orbital floor, showing orbital fat prolapsed into the maxillary antrum and the inferior rectus muscle adjacent to the fracture.
b. Sagittal CT scan of an orbital floor blow-out fracture, showing orbital fat prolapsed into the maxillary antrum below the inferior rectus muscle.

Radiological investigation

1. Plain X-rays may show blood within the antrum, and prolapse of orbital contents through the roof of the antrum (tear drop sign).

2. CT scans with direct coronal views are the best means of diagnosing orbital floor and medial wall fractures, showing their exact site and extent and the amount of prolapsed orbital tissue (Fig. 8.1).

Surgical repair of orbital floor fractures

Principle
The fracture is defined, prolapsed orbital contents repositioned, and the fracture reduced, with or without an implant or bone graft.

Indications
This is a controversial issue. There are those who believe no surgery is required for the fracture, and any squint is treated later on its merits.

Others operate on all blow-out fractures. A middle road is probably appropriate, and the following are generally accepted as indications to operate.

1. Diplopia persisting beyond a week to ten days and occurring in the primary position, reading position (down gaze), or in up gaze if occupation or recreation demands single vision in this position.

2. Large fractures with prolapse of considerable amounts of orbital fat likely to lead to significant enophthalmos (more than 2 mm). This is a relative indication, and is dependent on patient concerns about cosmetic appearance.

3. Infraorbital nerve paraesthesia alone is not an indication to operate, and this usually recovers spontaneously. Rare cases of persistent dysaesthesia due to compression of the infraorbital nerve by bone fragments or fibrous tissue may justify late decompression of the nerve in its canal.

Methods

1. Direct approach
2. Transconjunctival approach
3. Subciliary approach.

1. Direct approach
    a. Perform a forced duction test to gauge muscle restriction. Place a transconjunctival 4/0 silk traction suture under the tendon of the inferior rectus (Fig. 8.2). This aids in delineating entrapped tissue that has direct or indirect attachments to the inferior rectus and its sheath.
    b. Make a skin incision sloping across the orbital rim, within a skin fold if present (Fig. 8.3).
    c. Divide the orbicularis, or separate its fibres if in the line of the incision.
    d. Expose the inferior orbital rim.
    e. Incise the periosteum just outside the orbit (Fig. 8.4), and elevate it towards the floor of the orbit.
    f. Once on the floor of the orbit, the periorbita elevates easily. The fracture is usually on the medial side of the infraorbital canal. Locate the fracture and define its extent – this is made easier by dissecting along the extraperiosteal plane where the bone is intact, and approaching the fracture this way. It is important also

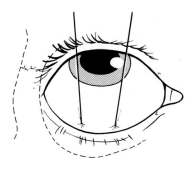

Fig. 8.2. Orbital floor fracture repair. Inferior rectus bridle suture.

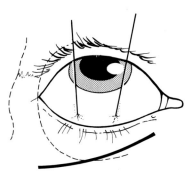

Fig. 8.3. Inferior skin incision.

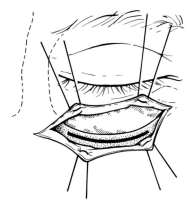

Fig. 8.4. Periosteal incision over inferior orbital rim.

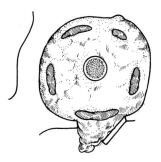

Fig. 8.5. Prolapsed contents of orbit through orbital floor fracture.

to delineate the posterior extent of the fracture. Remember that a floor fracture cannot extend beyond its junction with the posterior wall of the antrum, and this is a useful landmark once the antrum is entered.

g. Reposition any prolapsed orbital contents into the orbit. This may be difficult if a linear fracture has entrapped tissue within it, or if the fracture has been present for more than a few weeks. It may be necessary to depress the fracture further to enable the contents to be repositioned (Fig. 8.5). Hold the prolapsed fat within the orbit with a broad malleable retractor.

h. Redefine the site and extent of the fracture, and make sure its posterior limit has been reached. If a linear fracture is present without significant displacement, no implant may be required.

i. If there is depression of a hinged fragment of bone, reposition it

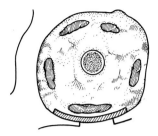

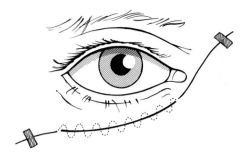

Fig. 8.6. Implant placed across fracture site.

Fig. 8.7. Wound closure.

if possible and hold it in place with a wedge of bone fragment or foreign sheet implant.

j. If a defect exists and inadequate bone is present to fill the gap, or it is too comminuted, an implant or bone graft is placed in the orbital floor (Fig. 8.6), supported on intact ledges of bone where they exist.

k. Any implant should be rigid enough to support the orbital contents; otherwise, the antrum can be packed from below via an antrostomy. Bone grafts can be harvested from the anterior maxillary wall, the outer table of the skull or the inner plate of the angle of the mandible, or nasal septal cartilage can be used. Iliac crest is usually not required except for very large and depressed fractures, and it may need to be plated in position.

l. Suture the periosteum over the orbital rim with 4/0 chromic catgut or longer acting absorbable interrupted sutures. Close the wound in two layers with 5/0 chromic catgut and 6/0 sub-cuticular nylon (Fig. 8.7).

2. Transconjunctival approach

a. Make a lateral canthotomy, sloping inferiorly (Fig. 8.8).

b. Using blunt scissors, open the plane between orbicularis and orbital septum. Incise the conjunctiva, fused retractors and orbital septum at the inferior border of the tarsus (Fig. 8.9), and then dissect in a plane between the orbital septum and the posterior surface of the orbicularis muscle to the orbital rim.

c. Expose the orbital rim (Fig. 8.10) and proceed as above.

d. Close the conjunctiva and retractors with interrupted or continuous 6/0 catgut suture (Fig. 8.11).

e. Reinsert the lateral canthal tendon inside the orbital rim using a long acting absorbable 5/0 suture.

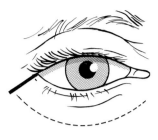

Fig. 8.8. Inferior fornix approach to orbital floor fracture, lateral canthotomy.

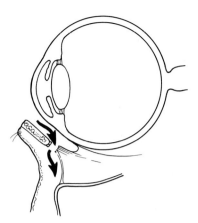

Fig. 8.9. Incision below tarsal plate through septum and lower lid retractors.

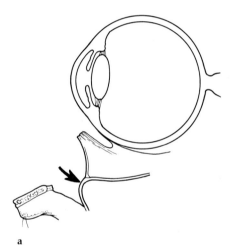

a

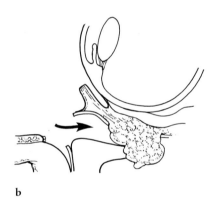

b

Fig. 8.10 a. Incision through periosteum on orbital rim. **b.** Periorbita elevated and fracture site approached.

    f. Close the canthotomy with 6/0 long acting absorbable sutures to the muscle, and 6/0 silk or nylon to the skin. Take care to reform the canthal angle.

3. Subciliary approach

    a. Make a subciliary skin incision and extend it laterally (Fig. 8.12).

    b. Raise the skin flap towards the orbital rim (Fig. 8.13a). Alternatively, the incision may be deepened through the orbicularis and dissection can proceed in the plane between the orbital septum and orbicularis to the inferior orbital rim (as above) (Fig. 8.14a, b).

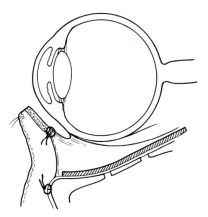

Fig. 8.11. Implant across fracture site and periosteum and conjunctiva closed.

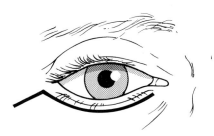

Fig. 8.12. Subciliary incision.

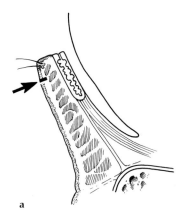

a

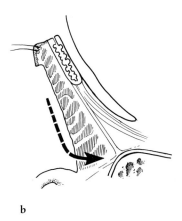

b

Fig. 8.13 a. Skin incision. **b**. Skin flap raised, orbicularis divided and orbital rim approached.

c. Divide the orbicularis over the inferior orbital rim (Fig. 8.13b) and proceed as above.

d. Close the muscle with 5/0 chromic catgut and the skin with a continuous 6/0 nylon (Fig. 8.15).

MEDIAL WALL FRACTURES

If a significant medial wall fracture is present, especially with entrapment of the medial rectus muscle or its attachments (Fig. 8.16), causing horizontal diplopia, it should be explored and repaired using the same principles as for a floor fracture.

The medial wall can sometimes be adequately exposed by any of the approaches outlined above, extending the dissection up the medial

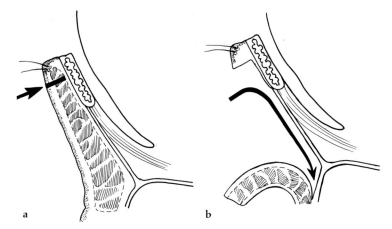

Fig. 8.14 a. Subciliary incision through skin and orbicularis. **b.** Skin and muscle flap raised and orbital rim exposed.

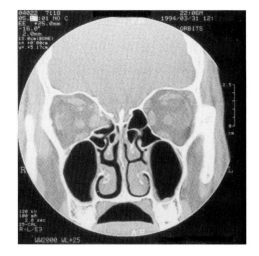

Fig. 8.15. Wound closed.

Fig. 8.16. A coronal CT of a right medial blow-out fracture. The patient had limited abduction and adduction of the right globe.

orbital wall. A better exposure may be obtained by using a separate medial skin incision or a medial conjunctival incision as outlined in Chapter 7 (Orbital Decompression), or by a coronal incision.

Complications

1. *Persistent diplopia.* This is common. After waiting for any spontaneous recovery over a six month period and a subsequent period of stability, squint surgery can be undertaken.

2. *Persistent enophthalmos.* This occurs if an inadequate reduction of the fracture has occurred, if any bone graft has resorbed, or if a medial or lateral wall fracture has been missed or left untreated. If cosmetically

significant, the fracture may be re-explored and bone grafts placed to overcome the deformity.

3. *Infection of a foreign implant or bone graft.* This is surprisingly rare. If it occurs after several weeks, an implant can be removed and no further treatment of the fracture is usually required, as dense fibrosis around the implant is usually adequate to support the contents of the orbit. If it occurs early, and does not settle with parenteral antibiotics, the implant should be removed. An infected bone graft usually resorbs. Later bone grafting may be required once infection has settled.

4. *Blindness.* This is rare, and is caused by swelling and/or haemorrhage compromising the circulation to the optic nerve or retina. Because of this risk, vision should be carefully monitored postoperatively. If vision deteriorates, the wound may need to be reopened, clot evacuated and any implant or bone graft removed. Steroids may reduce oedema.

5. *Lower eyelid malposition.* Lower lid retraction may occur if the orbital septum or orbicularis muscle is traumatized, and scars. Release of any scar tissue and a formal recession of the lower lid retractors with a spacer graft may then be required. Trasnconjunctival approaches may result in entropion if the conjunctival wound is sutured in such a way as to shorten the posterior lamella. Ectropion may occur with subciliary incisions, or if a lateral canthotomy is not carefully repaired.

Orbital haemorrhage

Orbital haemorrhage may complicate orbital fractures or blunt or penetrating orbital trauma without fractures. Spontaneous orbital haemorrhage may also occur in patients with vascular anomalies of the orbit, most usually in the venous/lymphangioma spectrum. If the haemorrhage is causing a rise in orbital pressure to the point where vision is compromised, this pressure may be relieved by one or more of the following measures.

1. *Lateral canthal release.* Make a straight lateral canthotomy incision for about 1 cm, deepening it to the periosteum over the lateral orbital rim (Fig. 8.17a). Grasp the lower eyelid and feel for the lower limb of the lateral canthal tendon with scissors, and divide it so that the lower lid is now mobile. With blunt-tipped scissors, use this wound to divide the lateral portion of the inferior orbital septum and lower

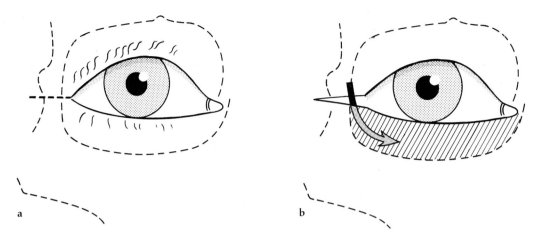

Fig. 8.17 a. A lateral cantholysis incision (dotted line).
b. Extension of the lateral canthal release (arrow) to divide the lower limb of the lateral canthal tendon and the lateral orbital septum.

eyelid retractors to further mobilize the lower eyelid and relieve the intraorbital pressure (Fig. 8.17b).

2. *Systemic corticosteroids and osmotic agents.* High dose steroids may help reduce orbital oedema. Osmotic agents given intravenously may also assist.

3. *Reduction of intraocular pressure.* This may increase retinal and optic disc perfusion. Anterior chamber paracentesis provides the most rapid and dramatic reduction, but intravenous acetazolamide, osmotic agents and topical pressure-lowering agents may also be used.

4. *Urgent orbital decompression.* Decompression of the orbital floor (if not already fractured) or medial wall may reduce orbital pressure if there is a diffuse intraorbital haemorrhage. Opening the orbital septum of the upper and lower eyelids through eyelid crease incisions may also help.

5. *Drainage of haematoma.* Most cases do not have a haematoma that is sufficiently localized for drainage to be possible. Occasionally, a large haematoma may collect in the extraperiosteal space and require urgent drainage or aspiration. A CT scan is needed to diagnose this.

Traumatic optic neuropathy

Optic neuropathy secondary to trauma may be due to a direct penetrating injury, tractional and deceleration forces (sometimes resulting in partial or complete avulsion of the optic nerve from the globe), pressure from orbital haemorrhage and oedema, haemorrhage and oedema within the optic nerve sheath or optic canal, or fractures of the optic canal. Intracranial optic nerve injury may also occur.

Optic neuropathy secondary to raised orbital pressure from haemorrhage or oedema should be managed as above. Haemorrhage within the optic nerve sheath may (rarely) cause deteriorating vision and require optic nerve sheath fenestration (see Chapter 4). Direct optic nerve trauma or avulsion is not amenable to treatment.

Controversy surrounds the management of traumatic optic neuropathy with an apparently anatomically intact optic nerve or an optic canal fracture. Most agree that high-dose corticosteroids may help reduce optic nerve oedema, and possibly reduce further optic nerve fibre loss or even salvage some reversibly damaged fibres. The place of optic nerve decompression is unclear. Some advocate decompression of the optic canal, especially where a fracture is present or a fragment of bone appears to be impinging on the nerve. This decompression may be achieved through a transnasal endoscopic approach, removing bone from the medial wall of the optic canal in the lateral wall of the sphenoid sinus, with or without direct exposure, via a medial extraperiosteal anterior orbitotomy or transcranially. Whether this alters the natural outcome in these patients is unknown.

Further reading

Dutton, J. (1991). Management of blow-out fractures of the orbital floor. *Surv. Ophthalmol.*, **35**, 279–298.

Jordan, D. R., Onge, P. S., Anderson, R. L. *et al.* (1992). Complications of alloplastic implants used in orbital fracture repair. *Ophthalmology*, **99**, 1600–1608.

Westfall, C. T., Shore, J. W., Nunery, W. R. *et al.* (1991). Operative complications of the transconjunctival inferior fornix approach. *Ophthalmology*, **98**, 1525–1528.

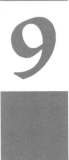

9

Orbital infection and foreign bodies

Surgery forms a small but important part of the management of orbital infection. In orbital cellulitis, surgery may be required for the treatment of underlying sinus disease or drainage of an orbital abscess. ENT surgeons should manage the sinus disease, but ophthalmologists should take a central role in the management of orbital cellulitis because visual loss may occur quite rapidly or suddenly, even whilst parenteral antibiotic therapy is underway. Careful monitoring of the vision is mandatory.

Diagnosis

The signs of orbital cellulitis are:

1. Fever, local pain, lid swelling and erythema

2. Conjunctival chemosis

3. Restricted eye movements

4. Proptosis

5. Reduced vision.

Any of the symptoms (2) to (5) above may be present. If all of them are absent, then the cellulitis is confined to the eyelids and the patient has preseptal cellulitis by definition. Orbital cellulitis most often occurs in a child or young adult with a history of sinus disease. Admission to hospital is mandatory. The following steps should be taken:

1. Try to establish the causative organism. The most likely source of positive cultures is pus from within the sinuses or their draining ostia, which ENT surgeons can retrieve for culture. Blood cultures may also occasionally be positive. Conjunctival and nasal swabs are usually negative or non-contributory.

2. Commence appropriate high-dose, broad-spectrum parenteral anti-

biotics in consultation with the microbiologists. Perform an urgent CT scan of the orbits and anterior cranial fossa and sinuses as a baseline.

3. Monitor signs of infection for improvement or deterioration, and chart them. This includes visual acuity, pupil responses (looking for an afferent defect), eye movements, proptosis, chemosis and lid swelling.

4. If there is a deterioration in vision or no improvement after an initial response to antibiotics, consider the possibility of an orbital abscess. Repeat the CT scan. If no abscess is seen, reducing orbital pressure by a lateral cantholysis may help (see Chapter 8), high-dose steroids may reduce oedema, and an external ethmoidectomy may partially decompress the orbit whilst treating the underlying cause. If an abscess is present, it should be drained urgently. The commonest site is the subperiosteal plane on the medial orbital wall.

Drainage of subperiosteal abscess (Fig. 9.1)

1. Make a vertical incision midway between the medial canthus and the midline (Fig. 9.2). Deepen it to the periosteum.

2. Incise the periosteum and elevate it to expose the bone anterior to the lacrimal crest. Continue the periosteal elevation beyond the anterior lacrimal crest, elevating the lacrimal sac out of its fossa and

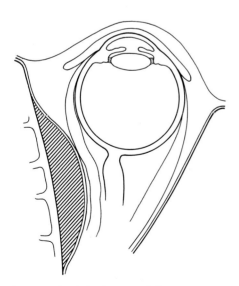

Fig. 9.1. Medial subperiosteal abscess.

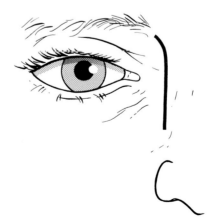

Fig. 9.2. Incision for drainage of abscess.

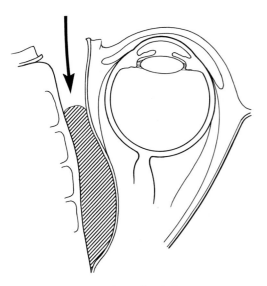

Fig. 9.3. Periosteum elevated and abscess cavity approached.

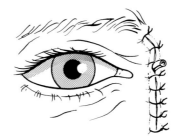

Fig. 9.4. Wound closed with drain tube in place.

exposing the medial wall of the orbit. If an abscess is present, pus will appear in the wound (Fig. 9.3).

3. It should be collected for Gram stain, culture and sensitivities.

4. All pus is sucked out, and the abscess cavity thoroughly explored to break down any other loculi.

5. If an external ethmoidectomy is required, it can be done through this incision.

6. Place a drain tube in the cavity, and close the wound in layers (Fig. 9.4).

7. The drain is removed when pus no longer drains, or after several days (when the track should remain open) if pus is still draining.

Other orbital abscesses

If an abscess occurs elsewhere in the orbit, the most direct surgical approach possible is made in order to to minimize trauma to important structures. Bone should not need to be removed, and direct approaches via the extraperiosteal space or lid are adequate. Another common site for an abscess complicating sinus infection is in the upper eyelid and brow, with or without extension into the superior subperiosteal space, in association with a frontal sinus infection. There is often a defect in the bone of the floor of the frontal sinus.

Rhino-orbital mucormycosis

This rare but often fatal fungal infection occurs in poorly controlled diabetics often in ketoacidosis, and in immunocompromised (but not AIDS) patients. It has increasingly been seen in renal dialysis patients and others on the iron- and aluminium-chelating agent, desferrioxamine. Early diagnosis and aggressive treatment is important if the patient is to survive.

It presents as a sinus and orbital infection, which may progress to necrosis of skin (eschar formation) or mucous membrane and underlying tissue by causing thrombosis and obliteration of blood vessels. If rhino-orbital mucormycosis is suspected, the following steps are required:

1. Obtain tissue for immediate microscopic examination and culture. The microbiologist should be warned of the suspected diagnosis, as special techniques may be required to identify the fungus. Tissue can be obtained from affected sinuses or from the orbit.
2. If confirmed, immediate surgery is required to excise all affected tissue. This often means orbital exenteration plus radical sinus surgery. Systemic antifungal agents are commenced. Even with these measures, there is a high mortality rate.

Orbital foreign bodies

A variety of foreign bodies may enter the orbit, and not all need to be removed. A common foreign body is a pellet fired by a small-bore airgun, to which children are unfortunately often allowed access. These do not need to be removed from the orbit unless they are impinging on the periorbita and causing pain. Infection and other sequelae are rare.

Foreign bodies made of organic material such as wood must be removed, as infection with a discharging sinus is inevitable.

Any patient with a history of a penetrating orbital injury should be suspected of having a foreign body, and thorough radiological investigation undertaken. The possibility of penetration of the cranial cavity should also be borne in mind. Wood may not show up well on CT scans, and MRI, if available, may be required to demonstrate it.

10

Diagnosis and investigation of lacrimal disease

History and examination

In most patients with lacrimal excretory system disease a diagnosis can be established on the basis of history and examination, without resort to any sophisticated investigations. Imaging studies such as dacryocystography, CT (with or without contrast agents in the tear ducts) and MRI are not often necessary, but may serve as an adjunct. The only readily available functional study of tear excretion that supplements clinical examination is nuclear lacrimal scanning.

HISTORY

Patients with lacrimal excretory system disease present with a limited number of symptoms:

1. Epiphora, or a watering eye
2. Discharge
3. Swelling in the region of the lacrimal sac
4. Pain
5. Blurred vision
6. Fistula
7. Bleeding from the eye.

Each symptom is analysed carefully for its nature, severity and time relationships. Duration and time of onset of symptoms give important clues as to the cause.

Watering of the eye may occur due to increased secretion beyond the amount that the normal tear ducts can drain, or because of abnormalities in the tear drainage system. Physiological tearing occurs with emotional weeping or in cold windy conditions. Reflex hypersecretion may occur in response to irritation of the ocular surface by foreign bodies, ingrown eyelashes (trichiasis) or infection. An important cause of reflex watering is dry eye. If basal tear secretion and normal wetting of the ocular surface by blinking is inadequate to prevent punctate ulceration of the cornea or conjunctiva, reflex epiphora may occur in response to the surface ulceration. In these patients, watering is often worse in dry, warm conditions or when blinking is reduced (for example when concentrating on reading, driving, watching television or using a computer screen), or in conditions such as Parkinson's disease where blinking is infrequent. Infrequent or absent blinking (as in facial palsy) may cause drying of the ocular surface and reflex tearing, but also will reduce tear drainage by lacrimal pump failure.

The patient with reflex tearing due to surface drying contrasts with the patient with an anatomical or functional obstruction of the tear ducts, who finds that watering is worse in conditions that increase tear secretion, such as cold windy conditions.

The constancy of watering also gives a clue to aetiology. For example, an infant whose eye waters only in the presence of an upper respiratory infection is likely to have stenosis of the lower end of the nasolacrimal duct, rather than complete obstruction.

Discharge from the eye in association with watering usually indicates the presence of a mucocoele of the lacrimal sac, especially when the discharge increases with pressure over the lacrimal sac. Some patients with dry eye may have mucus accumulation.

A swollen lacrimal sac present from birth usually represents a dacryocoele or dacryops (see Chapter 11). Later onset usually indicates a mucocoele or pyocoele, and there will of course be painful swelling of the lacrimal sac and overlying tissues in the presence of acute dacryocystitis. Tumours of the lacrimal sac may also cause swelling, and these will be incompressible. Some lacrimal mucocoeles will also be incompressible, as the opening of the common canaliculus into the lacrimal sac may be obstructed by mucosal swelling, a membrane, or by a flap valve effect of the mucosa as the common canaliculus enters in an oblique direction.

Occasionally, a swollen lacrimal sac may be due to distension by air. Such distension may sometimes be painful, and then relieved suddenly by pressure over the sac as the air is expelled down the nasolacrimal duct.

Other than acute distension of the lacrimal sac, which may also occur in the presence of a lacrimal stone (see Chapter 12), the usual cause of pain and tenderness in the region of the lacrimal sac is acute infection (dacryocystitis).

Patients with watery eyes often complain of blurred vision. This is usually worse with reading, because in down gaze the enlarged tear meniscus distorts the image entering the pupil. Blurring may also be due to mucus in the tear film, and repeated blinking usually clears this.

Some patients will notice a lacrimal fistula, but often it goes unnoticed. If its presence dates from birth, it is clearly congenital. Fistulae occurring after an episode of acute dacryocystitis or drainage of a lacrimal sac abscess are acquired. The management of these different types of fistulae is described in Chapter 12.

Bleeding from the eye, or bloody tears, is a rare but important symptom and should alert the examiner to the possibility of malignancy of the lacrimal excretory system. However, other conditions can also cause bleeding, including inflammation of the lacrimal sac or pyogenic granulomas of the sac or canaliculi, the latter often seen in canaliculitis. Psychiatrically disturbed patients may also inflict trauma upon themselves, causing bleeding.

EXAMINATION

A logical examination sequence will establish the presence and site of lacrimal obstruction in nearly all patients. The following steps are necessary:

1. Exclude causes of reflex tearing such as trichiasis, foreign body, punctate corneal ulceration from dry eye, etc. Observe the frequency of blinking.

2. Make sure the lacrimal puncta are normal and in a position to accept tears, not ectropic, closed over by membranes or entirely absent. Stenosis of the puncta has to be very severe to cause watering, and enlarging them by a traditional 3-snip operation will often reduce the functional ability of the canaliculus to drain tears.

3. Assess the horizontal laxity of the lid. Severe laxity may reduce the lacrimal pump mechanism, and simple lid tightening may improve symptoms.

4. Palpate and massage the lacrimal sac, for the presence of a mucocoele or tumour.

5. Syringe the lacrimal system. A fine, gently curved lacrimal cannula (26 gauge) should be used, and the punctum does not usually need to be dilated. Place the cannula several millimetres into the inferior canaliculus, syringe some fluid through and observe where the fluid goes. This will give information about the level of any obstruction. The sac may be palpated during syringing, and if it dilates, the obstruction is below the sac.

6. If not patent, gently pass the cannula towards the sac (if possible) to determine the length of patent canaliculus, and measure it if the sac cannot be reached. The upper canaliculus may be syringed and probed, but only if the lower canaliculus does not communicate with it as evidenced by reflux of fluid via the upper punctum on syringing.

7. If the system is patent, dye tests can be performed to see if the obstruction is a functional one.

8. Fluorescein dye is instilled into the conjunctival sac, and after five minutes the patient's nose is blown onto a white tissue. If no dye appears, a fine cotton-tipped applicator is placed under the inferior turbinate to see if dye has passed into the nose. If this is negative, plain saline is syringed through the system. If dye appears in the nose, it indicates that tears have drained at least as far as the lacrimal sac.

9. The rate of disappearance of fluorescein-stained tears may be semiquantitatively assessed, and a comparison made between the two sides. This dye disappearance test is useful in young children and infants.

10. Examine the patient's nasal cavity with a head light and nasal speculum. This important step helps to exclude the possibility of tumours obstructing the nasolacrimal duct and aids in planning the surgery, as a nasal airway is essential through which to drain the tears via a dacryocystorhinostomy, and an adequate space is required in those patients needing a lacrimal bypass tube. A nasal endoscope is useful for assessing nasal disease more thoroughly, and is also helpful in assessing postoperative patients.

SPECIAL INVESTIGATIONS

1. Dacryocystography
2. CT scan
3. CT and dacryocystography
4. Nuclear lacrimal scanning.

Dacryocystography

Dacryocystography (DCG) is performed by injecting radio-opaque dye into one canaliculus and taking X-rays whilst injecting. Films are taken with the patient supine. Additional information can be obtained by performing delayed erect films (10–15 minutes later) to see how well

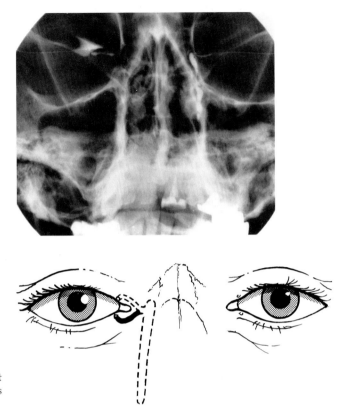

Fig. 10.1. There is an obstruction at the distal end of the inferior canaliculus on the right side.

the tear duct empties. This gives some information on the function of the tear ducts. It is always useful to compare both sides.

DCGs give additional information on the anatomy of the canaliculi, lacrimal sac and nasolacrimal duct (Figs 10.1–10.4). Although a DCG is not necessary when planning lacrimal surgery, it may be impossible to clinically differentiate an obstruction with a small sac from a common canalicular obstruction without it. A DCG is also helpful in assessing the patient with epiphora and a patent lacrimal system. By comparing the two sides and performing delayed erect films, stenoses and poor emptying may be detected. DCGs may also detect stones (Fig. 10.4) or lacrimal sac tumours, and are invaluable in assessing a patient after a failed dacryocystorhinostomy (DCR).

CT scanning

CT scans give information about the bony and soft tissue anatomy in the region of the lacrimal sac and nasolacrimal duct that is not seen with DCG. They are useful if there is any suspicion of tumours impinging on or involving the lacrimal sac or nasolacrimal duct, and are helpful in

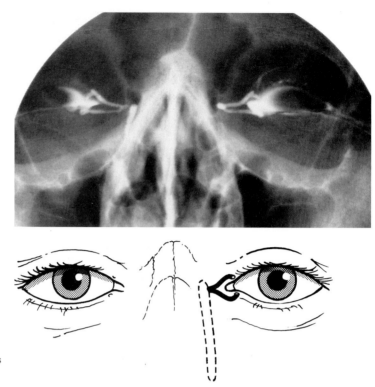

Fig. 10.2. The common canaliculus is obstructed on the left.

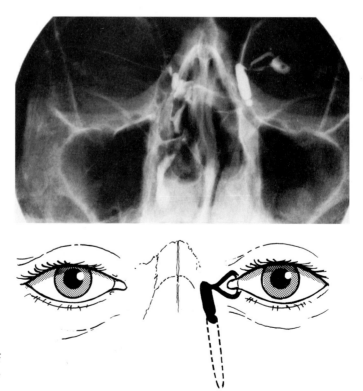

Fig. 10.3. There is an obstruction of the lower end of the left lacrimal sac, which is dilated.

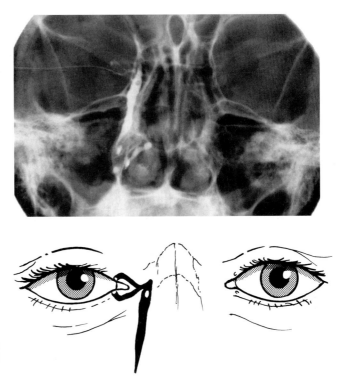

Fig. 10.4. A filling defect due to a small dacryolith is present in the lacrimal sac.

assessing the anatomy in patients after failed DCR. They also help in planning lacrimal surgery in patients with facial fractures or craniofacial anomalies, remembering that it is of course necessary to have a nasal airway medial to the lacrimal sac and upper nasolacrimal duct in order to perform a DCR.

CT scanning with dacryocystography

The presence of radio-opaque dye in the lacrimal sac and nasolacrimal duct helps further to define the anatomy of the lacrimal excretory system, both before surgery and after failed surgery.

Nuclear lacrimal scanning

This technique (also called lacrimal scintigraphy) is the best current method to assess functional tear drainage. A drop of radioactively labelled fluid is placed in each eye, and the tear drainage followed over time with a gamma camera. The anatomical level reached and the time required to reach that point can be determined. However, anatomical detail is not well shown, with poor resolution of the images.

Further reading

Hurwitz, J. J. (1996). *The Lacrimal System*. Lippincott-Raven.

Welham, R. A. (1989). Lacrimal surgery. In *A Manual of Systematic Eyelid Surgery* (J. R. O. Collin, ed.). pp. 109–120. Churchill Livingstone.

11

Congenital lacrimal obstruction

Congenital lacrimal obstruction is common, and nearly all cases are due to failure of complete canalization of the lower end of the nasolacrimal duct (Fig. 11.1). Most cases resolve in the first 10 months of life, and a much smaller percentage after that. Many surgeons would elect to intervene between 6 and 12 months if symptoms of watering and discharge persist, or earlier if dacryocystitis supervenes (which is rare). Many cases will still resolve between 6 and 10 months of age, so intervention may be delayed until 10 months. Massage of the lacrimal sac may hasten spontaneous resolution.

A small number of infants are born with a tense swelling of the lacrimal sac known as a dacryocoele. It results from obstruction at the upper and lower ends of the drainage system, probably with a flap valve effect at the internal common punctum preventing escape of fluid onto the eye, and most resolve spontaneously in the first weeks of life. Dacryocystitis may supervene and probing may be required early. Some have a cystic enlargement of the lower end of the nasolacrimal duct presenting below the inferior turbinate, which may obstruct the nasal airway.

Lacrimal probing

Principle
A metal probe is passed down the lacrimal drainage system to overcome an obstruction at the lower end.

Indications

1. Persistent watering and discharge after the age of 10 months

2. Dacryocystitis.

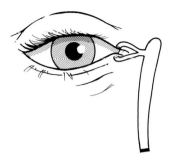

Fig. 11.1. Site of congenital lacrimal obstruction.

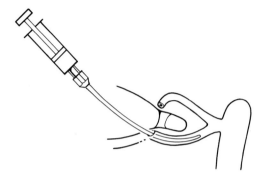

Fig. 11.2. Lacrimal cannula inserted in the inferior canaliculus for syringing.

Method

1. Dilate a punctum and pass a lacrimal cannula vertically into the first 2 mm of the canaliculus, and then horizontally for several millimetres (Fig. 11.2). Syringe some fluorescein-stained saline into the lacrimal system, and observe whether it refluxes or passes into the nose, where it can be sucked out with a fine catheter. This simple manoeuvre may be enough to overcome thin membranous obstructions or demonstrate a patent system.

2. If fluid does not pass into the nose, exchange the cannula for a fine 0 or 2/0 probe. Maintaining traction on the lid to keep the canaliculus straight, pass the probe into the lacrimal sac until a hard stop is felt as the tip of the probe reaches the medial wall of the sac (Fig. 11.3a, b, c).

3. Swing the probe vertically to pass down the nasolacrimal duct (Fig.11.3d). Its direction is not absolutely vertical, having a slight posterior and medial slant. A sense of a membrane giving way will usually be felt at the lower end as the nose is entered (Fig. 11.3e).

4. Pass the cannula into the sac again, and inject some fluid or air to determine the patency of the system.

5. If the first probing does not create a patent system, the inferior turbinate can be infractured (Fig. 11.3f) and the probing repeated.

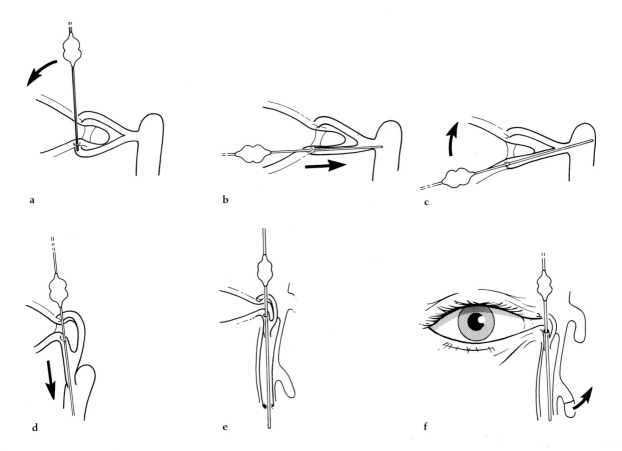

Fig. 11.3 a. Lacrimal probe inserted vertically into the punctum and first part of the canaliculus.
b. The probe swung horizontally and passed into the lacrimal sac.
c. The probe swung vertically with the tip against the medial wall of the sac.
d. The probe passed down the nasolacrimal duct.
e. The probe passes the membranous obstruction into the nose.
f. The inferior turbinate is fractured medially.

Placing the cannula vertically in the nasolacrimal duct whilst syringing may also more readily demonstrate patency than placing it in the canaliculus.

Complications

1. *Bleeding.* A small amount of bleeding is not uncommon.

2. *Failure to pass the probe.* Rarely, there is no bony nasolacrimal canal, and no hope of passing the probe. A DCR will be required.

3. *Failure of the symptoms to resolve.* In this situation, a repeat probing may be performed with infracture of the inferior turbinate, if not

already done. If this second probe fails, the options are lacrimal intubation or DCR.

Lacrimal intubation for congenital obstruction

This technique works for the majority of young infants and children in whom probings have failed. The success rate decreases with increasing age.

Principle
The lacrimal system is intubated with fine silicone tubing, which is tied in the nose and left in place for three to six months.

Indications

1. Congenital lacrimal obstruction not responding to simple probings on two occasions.
2. The repair of lacerated canaliculi (see Chapter 13).

Method 1

1. Place some cocaine-soaked ribbon gauze or cotton wool beneath the inferior turbinate.
2. Pass a probe (as above) to determine the presence of the nasolacrimal duct, and whether the nose can be reached.
3. Widely dilate the puncta.
4. Remove the nasal packing and infracture the inferior turbinate.
5. Place some fine silicone tubing over the end of a 3/0 or 4/0 probe or a long, blunt 25-gauge needle, and fold it back on itself (Fig. 11.4a).
6. Pass the probe or needle with the tubing into the canaliculus and down the nasolacrimal duct as for a probing (Fig. 11.4b, c).
7. Under direct vision (a nasal endoscope may help) or by palpation with a fine instrument, locate the probe and tubing under the inferior turbinate. Grasp the end of the probe and tubing firmly and gently remove the probe or needle whilst sliding the tubing off the end, holding it by the instrument in the nose. Pull the end of the tubing out of the nostril and secure it. (An alternative and popular technique is to use one of the manufactured lacrimal intubation systems, which have tubing attached to fine wire probes with hooks

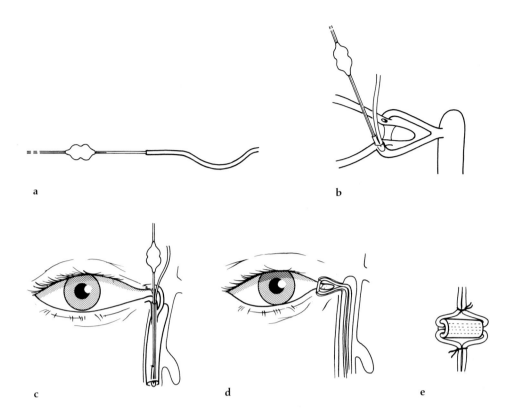

Fig. 11.4 a. Fine silicone tubing passed onto the end of a fine lacrimal probe (3/0).
b. The tubing bent back and the tip of the probe passed into the dilated punctum.
c. The probe and tubing passed down the nasolacrimal duct and retrieved from under the inferior turbinate.
d. Tubing passed similarly through the upper canaliculus.
e. The tubing secured in the nose to prevent prolapse onto the eye.

and guides designed for their retrieval. The whole system is pulled through the canaliculi and nasolacrimal duct and may unnecessarily traumatize the canaliculi and nose.)

8. Repeat the procedure in the opposite canaliculus with the other end of the tubing.

9. Tie the tubing in a knot or over a piece of heavier tubing reinforced above and below by a suture (Fig. 11.4d,e) or through a small piece of sponge, so that the tubing cannot escape up the nasolacrimal duct and out onto the eye. It should not be tied so tightly that the canaliculi will cheesewire through. The tubing may be secured to the lateral part of the nasal vestibule with a non-absorbable suture.

10. Remove the tubing via the nose three to six months later. This usually requires an anaesthetic. If the knot at the lower end is small enough to be pulled out through the canaliculi, it will not be large enough to prevent it from spontaneously prolapsing out.

Complications

1. *Cheesewiring of the canaliculi.* This should not occur if the tubing is not tied too tightly under the inferior turbinate.

2. *Granuloma formation.* This occasionally occurs at the punctum, and is removed at the same time as the tubing.

3. *Prolapse of the tubing onto the eye.* This is avoided by tying an adequate knot or piece of larger tubing under the inferior turbinate. An alternative method is to pass a nylon suture attached to the tube through the full thickness of the cartilaginous nasal septum, securing it on the other side.

4. *Persistent watering.* If due to genuine obstruction, a DCR will be required. Some infants with a patent system after probing or intubation will water intermittently, especially with an upper respiratory tract infection. This usually resolves as the child grows.

Further reading

Crawford, J. S. (1977). Intubation of obstructions of the lacrimal system. *Can. J. Ophthalmol.*, **12**, 289–292.

Henderson, P. N. and McNab, A. A. (1996). An alternative method of closed silicone intubation of the lacrimal system. *Ophthalmic Surg. Lasers*, **27**, 401–404.

MacEwen, C. J. and Young, J. D. H. (1991). Epiphora during the first year of life. *Eye*, **5**, 596–600.

Mansour, A. M., Cheng, K. P., Mumma, J. V. et al. (1991). Congenital dacryocoele. A collaborative review. *Ophthalmology*, **98**, 1744–1751.

12

Dacryocystorhinostomy

Dacryocystorhinostomy is the standard operation for lacrimal obstruction. It is indicated for anatomical obstructions, and may also help patients with a functional obstruction (an anatomically patent system that does not adequately drain tears).

As far as practicable, the level and cause of the obstruction should be established prior to surgery (see Chapter 10). Remember to ask for nasal symptoms, as occasionally patients with nasal and paranasal tumours will present with watering.

Choice of operation

The choice of operation is dependent on the level of the obstruction:

1. Obstruction within the nasolacrimal duct or junction of sac and duct: routine DCR, with or without tubes.
2. Obstruction at the internal common punctum (common canalicular obstruction): DCR and tubes.
3. Obstruction at or beyond 8 mm from the punctum of one or both canaliculi: canaliculo-DCR.
4. Obstruction less than 8 mm from the punctum in both canaliculi: DCR and bypass tube.

Haemostasis during lacrimal surgery

The key to lacrimal surgery is haemostasis. The following measures will help:

1. Place the patient head-up, and keep the blood pressure low.
2. Use local anaesthetic if feasible – blood loss is considerably less in locally anaesthetized patients, and the operation therefore more easily performed.
3. Spray and pack the nose with vasoconstrictors (local anaesthetics will also do this).

4. Dissect in tissue planes (avoids the angular vessels).

5. Use traction sutures (if placed full thickness from periosteum to skin, these will control bleeding from angular vessels if it occurs).

6. Place a sucker up the nose once the nasal mucosa is opened.

7. Suturing the flaps usually stops bleeding from the cut edges of the mucosa.

8. Use haemostatic agents such as thrombin-soaked sponges or cellulose sponges for persistent bleeding.

9. Packing the nose for persistent bleeding at the end of the procedure is rarely needed.

Dacryocystorhinostomy

Principle
A side-to-side anastomosis is made between the lacrimal sac and nasal cavity, effectively incorporating the lacrimal sac into the lateral wall of the nose (Fig. 12.1).

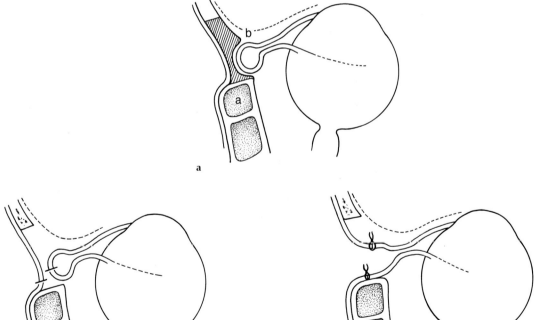

Fig. 12.1 a. Axial section of the lacrimal sac in its fossa to show the area of bone removed for DCR. a = anterior ethmoid air cell; b = anterior lacrimal crest.
b. Points of incision in the lacrimal sac and nasal mucosa (diagrammatic).
c. Side-to-side anastomosis between lacrimal sac and nasal mucosa.

Indications

1. Lacrimal mucocoele (obstruction at the sac and nasolacrimal duct junction).

2. Nasolacrimal duct obstruction in children not responding to probing and intubation, and nasolacrimal duct obstruction in adults.

3. Functional lacrimal obstruction not responding to simpler methods of treatment such as horizontal lid tightening.

Method

Local or general anaesthetic can be used. Bleeding tends to be less with local anaesthetic, but sedation is required. For both methods of anaesthesia, the nose is sprayed with a vasoconstrictor and local anaesthetic, and the middle meatus of the nose is then packed with ribbon gauze soaked in an anaesthetic such as cocaine. For local anaesthesia, the area of the medial canthus is infiltrated subcutaneously, the infraorbital nerve is blocked on the cheek and a medial peribulbar orbital injection via the caruncle is given to block the anterior ethmoidal and infratrochlear nerves.

1. Make an incision through the skin only, approximately 10 mm from the medial canthus on the side of the nose, starting several millimetres above the level of the canthus and extending in a straight line for about 3 cm towards the ala of the nose (Fig. 12.2).

2. Raise the skin from the underlying orbicularis and angular vessels, and place a traction stitch of 4/0 silk in each flap.

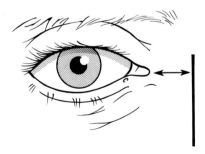

Fig. 12.2. Incision for DCR.

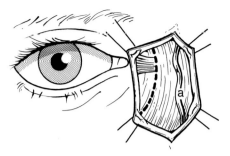

Fig. 12.3. Medial canthal tendon exposed. The angular vein (a) lies anteriorly on the orbicularis muscle. The orbicularis muscle is separated in the line of its fibres at the point of insertion of the canthal tendon (dotted line).

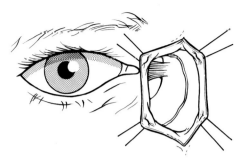

Fig. 12.4. The periosteum is incised and reflected anteriorly.

Fig. 12.5. The canthal tendon and periosteum are reflected laterally with the lacrimal sac to expose the lacrimal fossa.

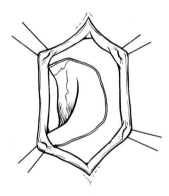

3. Locate the anterior limb of the medial canthal tendon (Fig. 12.3) and, at its point of insertion into the periosteum, separate the fibres of the orbicularis in their circumferential direction. This brings one to a point in front of the anterior lacrimal crest. Incise the periosteum in this line.

4. Elevate the periosteum anteriorly onto the nose for a centimetre or so (Fig. 12.4), then elevate it posteriorly, detaching the medial canthal tendon. Passing over the anterior lacrimal crest into the lacrimal fossa, reflect the whole of the lacrimal sac out of its fossa (Fig. 12.5).

5. Remove the nasal packing. This allows the nasal mucosa to be more easily pushed away from the inner aspect of the bone. Using a small right-angled elevator, force a hole in the thin bone at the junction of the lacrimal bone with the frontal process of the maxilla, in the centre or posterior third of the lacrimal fossa.

6. With the right-angled elevator, push the nasal mucosa away from the inner aspect of the bone.

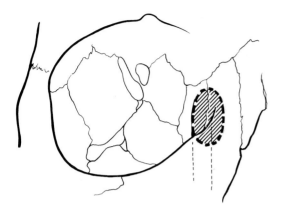

Fig. 12.6. The area of bone removed for DCR.

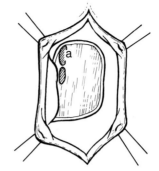

Fig. 12.7. The bony osteum formed. Anterior ethmoid cells posteriorly (a).

7. Outfracture a small piece of bone to allow the finest bone punch into the hole, and gradually enlarge the bony rhinostomy until the whole of the lacrimal fossa is removed, along with approximately 10 mm of bone anterior to the crest. The inferior limit should be level with the inferior orbital rim, and the first few millimetres of the medial wall of the bony nasolacrimal canal should also be taken (Figs 12.6 and 12.7). The superior limit should be 2–3 mm above the level of the entry of the common canaliculus into the lacrimal sac, so that no bone lies medial to the canaliculi.

8. An anterior ethmoidal air cell is often encountered when the rhinostomy is commenced. Its mucosa is much thinner than nasal mucosa. If in doubt, an instrument placed in the nose will help differentiate ethmoidal from nasal mucosa, with nasal mucosa moving with the movement of the instrument in the nose. If an ethmoidal air cell is encountered, continue making the rhinostomy anteriorly until the anterior edge of the air cell is reached. At this point it is necessary to force the right-angled elevator through the front wall of the air cell, bringing it between bone and nasal mucosa, and the rhinostomy is then enlarged in the usual way. Finally, remove any thin bone from the medial wall of the air cell to expose the full extent of the nasal mucosa.

9. Pass a probe into the sac. Where it tents up the mucosa of the medial wall of the sac (Fig. 12.8), make a vertical incision in the sac wall (Fig. 12.9) so that the end of the probe is visible. Enlarge this vertical opening in the sac for the full length of the sac and the first part of the nasolacrimal duct.

10. Make a vertical incision in the nasal mucosa (Fig. 12.9) to form

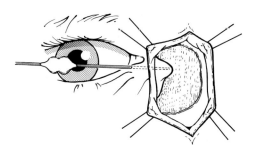

Fig. 12.8. A probe passed into the lacrimal sac.

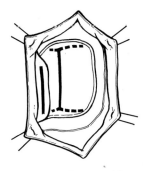

Fig. 12.9. The vertical lacrimal sac incision and the nasal mucosal incisions marked.

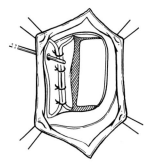

Fig. 12.10. The posterior mucosal flaps sutured with a probe in place.

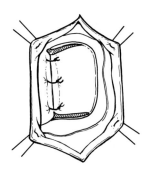

Fig. 12.11. The anterior mucosal flaps sutured.

anterior and posterior flaps, about two-thirds anterior, one-third posterior. It helps to place a broad flat instrument in the nose, such as a malleable retractor or flat scalpel handle, to protect the nasal septum and give something to cut against.

11. The posterior flap needs to be large enough to reach the posterior flap of the lacrimal sac, but not so large that it occludes the sac when folded outwards. It may sometimes need to be trimmed. Make relieving incisions above and below in the anterior flap to allow it to hinge forwards (Fig. 12.9). A 6/0 chromic catgut suture may be pre-placed at one corner and used to hold the anterior flap out of the way during suturing of the posterior flaps.

12. Place two or three interrupted sutures of 6/0 chromic catgut between the posterior sac and nasal flaps (Fig. 12.10). Using a half-circle needle, start within the sac, pick up the sac mucosa and then, with a separate bite, the nasal mucosa.

13. Suture the anterior flaps, again using 6/0 chromic catgut, with sufficient tension on the anterior flap to prevent it collapsing into the anastomosis (Fig. 12.11). Trim the anterior nasal flap if necessary to achieve this.

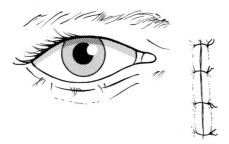

Fig. 12.12. The skin wound closed.

14. Re-approximate the anterior limb of the medial canthal tendon to the edge of the periosteum with 6/0 chromic catgut.

15. Close the skin with 6/0 nylon interrupted or subcuticular stitches (Fig. 12.12). Place a firm dressing over the area for 24 hours.

Complications

1. *Haemorrhage*

    a. *Intraoperatively.* Usually responds to the above measures. A nasal pack at the end of the procedure is rarely required.

    b. *Postoperatively.* A small amount of epistaxis is not uncommon. Larger haemorrhages do sometimes occur after several days, and are probably secondary to underlying infection. The nose may need to be packed and antibiotics given. Transfusion is rarely needed.

2. *Infection.* This is rare, and if it occurs, it usually means the operation has failed and there is obstruction with dacryocystitis. Parenteral antibiotics are required and the operation is repeated when the infection has settled.

3. *Persistent watering.* Scarring of the anastomosis with obstruction requires reoperation. Occasionally there is patency to syringing with persistent watering and discharge. In this situation, a sump syndrome may exist. The anastomosis is small and high up in the lacrimal sac. Tears and mucus accumulate in the sac and discharge onto the eye.

Dacryocystorhinostomy with tubes

Principle
A DCR is performed and the lacrimal canaliculi, common canaliculus, sac and anastomosis are stented postoperatively with fine silicone tubing.

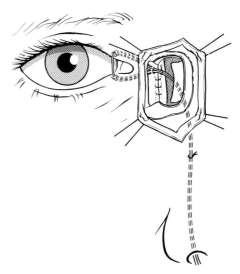

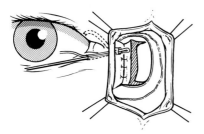

Fig. 12.13. Lacrimal tubing passed through the canaliculi on the end of a fine probe.

Fig. 12.14. Lacrimal tubing passed through both canaliculi and into the nose, and sutured together to prevent prolapse onto the eye.

Indications

1. A common canalicular obstruction
2. A small scarred lacrimal sac
3. Repeat DCR
4. Some surgeons routinely intubate all DCRs.

Method

1. Proceed as above until the lacrimal sac is opened. If a common canalicular obstruction is present, the probe will be prevented from entering the sac, usually by a thin membrane. Incising this carefully will allow the probe to enter the sac.

2. Intubate the canaliculi (Figs 12.13 and 12.14) and dilate the punctae. Pass fine silicone tubing over the end of a 3/0 or 4/0 probe or 26 gauge cannula, fold it back on itself, and pass the probe and tubing into the sac. Remove the tubing from the end of the probe. Repeat this in the opposite canaliculus with the other end of the tubing, and tie the two ends together with a 6/0 silk ligature 5–10 mm beyond the tube's exit from the common canaliculus so that the tubing cannot prolapse onto the eye. It should be tied so that a small loop of tubing lies loosely between the punctae without any tension. Drape the tubing back across the lids to help retract tissues and expose the posterior flaps for suturing.

3. Suture the posterior flaps. Pass a fine curved artery forcep up the nose, pass the two ends of the tubing into its jaws and pull the tubing out through the nose, trimming the ends at the nostril.

4. Complete the DCR as above.

5. Remove the tubing after two to three months, dividing it at the inner canthus and retrieving it through the nostril. When the patient's nose is blown, the tubing is brought to the nostril and a nasal speculum and head light (such as an indirect ophthalmoscope) helps in retrieving it from the nose.

Complications

1. If the tubing is tied too tightly, the canaliculi can be cheesewired by the tubing. If this begins to occur, the tubing is removed early.

2. Pyogenic granulomas may occur around the tubing at the puncta or at the site of the rhinostomy, especially if the tubing is left in place too long.

Repeat DCR

Principle
A previously failed DCR is revised to provide a patent anastomosis between the canaliculi, sac and nose.

Indications

1. Failed DCR with at least 8 mm of patent canaliculus.

2. Sump syndrome, with a patent but small high anastomosis in a dilated lacrimal sac full of tears and mucus.

Method
A preoperative dacryocystogram is useful in delineating the extent of patency, and helps in surgical planning. The same incision is used (Fig. 12.15), probes are placed in both canaliculi and skin flaps are raised and traction sutures placed in them.

1. Incise the scar tissue and periosteum over an area of bone away from the previous rhinostomy.

2. Expose a small area of bare bone by elevating the periosteum, and gradually enlarge this towards the rhinostomy until its edge is found.

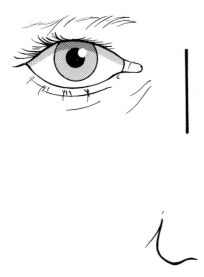

Fig. 12.15. Repeat DCR incision.

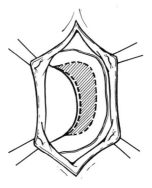

Fig. 12.16. The previous rhinostomy identified and enlarged.

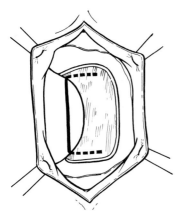

Fig. 12.17. A large anterior nasal mucosal flap is made.

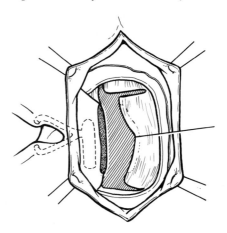

Fig. 12.18. The nasal mucosal flap retracted to show scar tissue across the old anastomosis.

3. Define the bony rhinostomy for 180 degrees or more of its circumference; this usually requires sharp dissection. Free the mucosa from the deep surface of the bone at the anterior edge of the old rhinostomy, and enlarge the rhinostomy for several millimetres around its exposed circumference or (if it is too small and in the wrong place) until its size and position are as for a primary DCR (Fig. 12.16).

4. Incise the nasal mucosa and old scarred anastomosis vertically (Fig. 12.17) and enter the nose with a sharp pointed blade to create a large anterior nasal flap (Fig. 12.18). The residual lacrimal sac is sometimes entered with this manoeuvre.

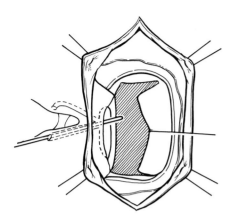

Fig. 12.19. A probe in the inferior canaliculus is revealed by progressive excision of scar tissue.

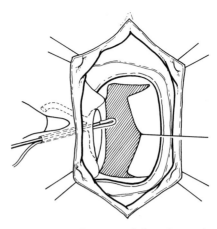

Fig. 12.20. Tubing passed through into the nose.

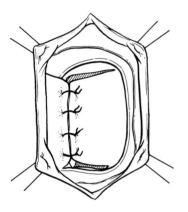

Fig. 12.21. The anterior mucosal flaps sutured.

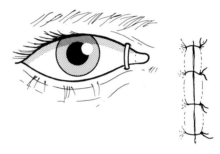

Fig. 12.22. The wound sutured.

5. With the probes in place, shave off successive layers of scar tissue until the ends of the probes are encountered and the residual sac opened (Fig. 12.19).

6. Open any residual lacrimal sac for its full vertical extent.

7. If posterior flaps can be manufactured, suture these. Often, a wall of scar tissue remains posteriorly.

8. Any posterior sac flap can be sutured back onto this.

9. Intubate the system (Fig. 12.20).

10. Suture the anterior flaps (Fig. 12.21) and skin (Fig. 12.22).

11. Remove the tubing after three months.

Sometimes it is possible to dissect the lacrimal sac and any scar tissue away from the old rhinostomy by sharply dissecting in the plane of the bone across the scarred rhinostomy until the full circumference of the old rhinostomy is outlined. The rhinostomy is then enlarged as appropriate, preserving the nasal mucosa with some scar tissue on its lateral aspect. This scar tissue may be trimmed once the nasal mucosal flaps are fashioned. The DCR is completed as for a primary DCR.

Miscellaneous lacrimal disorders

Several lacrimal disorders other than simple obstruction are encountered from time to time. These include:

1. Acute dacryocystitis
2. Canaliculitis
3. Lacrimal fistula – congenital or acquired
4. Dacryolithiasis (lacrimal stones)
5. Lacrimal sac tumours.

ACUTE DACRYOCYSTITIS

This occurs in the presence of lacrimal obstruction, usually at the junction of the sac and nasolacrimal duct, or (in children) from obstruction of the lower end of the nasolacrimal duct.

The presentation is commonly as follows:

1. There is usually a history of lacrimal obstruction – often for years.
2. There is a sudden onset over hours to days of a tender, red swelling over the medial canthus.
3. Fever and preseptal cellulitis may occur, and occasionally orbital cellulitis.
4. An abscess may develop within the lacrimal sac, and often extends outside the sac into the medial end of the lower lid. It will eventually point onto the skin, sometimes leading to a fistula.

Management

1. Admit to hospital.
2. Culture the conjunctiva, any discharge and any pus aspirated from the sac.
3. Commence parenteral antibiotics.
4. If an abscess is present, drain it. This is done with a wide-bore needle or a scalpel. Aspirating the lacrimal sac may relieve pain, and also provides material for microbiological examination. Any resultant

discharging fistula will close once the obstruction is relieved by subsequent surgery.

5. Once the acute infection has settled, proceed to DCR.

CANALICULITIS

This is an uncommon condition, which often goes undiagnosed for long periods. It is due to an infection within a canaliculus by streptothrix or actinomycetes organisms. The typical presentation is:

1. A purulent discharge from one punctum, with or without watering.
2. A red, slightly tender swelling over the canaliculus within the lid.
3. A bead of pus (with or without granules) appearing at the punctum with pressure over the canaliculus.
4. The punctum may have a pouting appearance, or a pyogenic granuloma may even protrude from it.
5. Patency to syringing through the canaliculus. Occasionally it is obstructed.
6. A very dilated canaliculus on dacryocystography, with multiple filling defects.

Management
This is simple and effective:

1. Dilate the punctum sufficiently to allow a small curette into the canaliculus. This may require a small vertical incision in the posterior wall of the vertical portion of the canaliculus.
2. Pass a curette into the canaliculus and scrape out the contents thoroughly. Typically, purulent material with yellowish granules is found.
3. If this fails to alleviate the symptoms, it can be repeated.
4. Alternatively, the canaliculus can be more widely opened along the portion within the lid margin, and the cavity curetted.
5. Antibiotics, either topically or systemically, will not cure the condition, but topical penicillin is sometimes given postoperatively.

LACRIMAL FISTULA

Congenital lacrimal fistulae
These are quite different from acquired fistulae, in that they are histologically like a normal canaliculus, with an epithelial lining. They

usually present in childhood, but occasionally remain asymptomatic into adulthood. The following features are seen:

1. The fistula usually opens onto the skin below the medial canthal tendon.
2. It often arises from the region of the common canaliculus, but can arise from the sac or even the NLD.
3. The canaliculi may be anatomically normal, or one or both may be partially or totally absent.
4. Watering is the usual presentation. Dacryocystitis or inflammation of the fistula may occur.
5. The patient may be aware of tears or mucus appearing on the skin at the mouth of the fistula.

Management
If symptomatic, the fistula is excised for its whole length and any underlying obstruction is treated on its merits.

Method

1. Place a fine probe in the fistula and one canaliculus.
2. Excise a small ellipse of skin around the mouth of the fistula and dissect it down towards its origin at the common canaliculus.
3. Tie a long acting absorbable suture around the base of the fistula, with the probe in the canaliculus protecting it.
4. Excise the fistula and close the skin.
5. If there is concern about the patency of the common canaliculus in a young child, or an associated lower obstruction, the system is intubated for three months.
6. If there is an associated lacrimal obstruction in an older child or adult, a DCR with tubes is performed.

Acquired lacrimal fistulae
These usually occur as the result of trauma to the canaliculi, or dacryocystitis. If there is underlying canalicular obstruction, the usual formula for choice of operation is followed.

Management
For a fistula complicating dacryocystitis, the management is:

1. Treat the acute dacryocystitis.

2. Perform a DCR.

The mouth of the fistula may be ignored, or it can be cauterized if granulations are present. It may be excised and sutured, but it is not necessary to excise its whole length as it is not epithelially lined and will close once the distal obstruction is overcome by the DCR.

DACRYOLITHIASIS

Lacrimal stones are not uncommon, and they may be small but can become large and form a cast of the lacrimal sac and upper nasolacrimal duct. The following features are typical:

1. The patient is usually a young or middle-aged adult woman.
2. Symptoms are often intermittent, with watering, some discharge, and (sometimes) a tense painful swelling of the lacrimal sac which may resolve suddenly with relief of symptoms.
3. Patency to syringing, often with some reflux of fluid.
4. A filling defect on dacryocystography.

The treatment is DCR and removal of the stone.

LACRIMAL SAC TUMOURS

These are rare. A variety of neoplasms may affect the lacrimal sac, but most are epithelial, including papilloma, transitional cell carcinoma and squamous cell carcinoma. Some are associated with human papilloma virus infection. Some tumours of the nose and paranasal sinuses may secondarily involve the lacrimal sac or nasolacrimal duct, and medial canthal cutaneous tumours may also invade this area.

Patients present with one or more of the following symptoms:

1. Epiphora
2. Bloody tears
3. Epistaxis or nasal discharge
4. A lump in the region of the lacrimal sac
5. Dacryocystitis.

A tumour in the lacrimal sac will give a non-compressible swelling of the sac. Sometimes a tense mucocoele will mimic this and be non-compressible. Aspirating the lacrimal sac with a large-bore needle will help to differentiate the two. On dacryocystography, a filling defect is seen in the sac, with or without bone destruction. A CT scan or MRI is helpful in planning treatment.

Unless the tumour is intraepithelial or benign, a radical dacryocystectomy is performed. This entails *en bloc* excision of the sac, nasolacrimal duct and surrounding bone, which by definition will include part of the medial wall of the orbit and the lateral wall of the nose and the inferior turbinate. The medial ends of the entire lacrimal canaliculi and medial lids and other canthal structures may also need to be excised to gain an adequate surgical margin when a malignant tumour occupies the lacrimal sac.

For intraepithelial malignancy (carcinoma in situ, papilloma with dysplasia, inverting papilloma), a less radical dacryocystectomy may be performed, with removal of the nasolacrimal duct as well if indicated. Dacryocystectomy has no place in the management of obstruction due to benign causes, and a DCR is more easily performed. The practice of performing dacryocystectomy in elderly or debilitated patients with simple obstruction is to be avoided. Occasionally, if a patient has a very dry eye, this may be justified when infection of the lacrimal sac is the indication.

Further reading

Hornblass, A., Jakobiec, F. A., Bosniak, S. and Flanagan, J. C. (1980). The diagnosis and management of epithelial tumors of the lacrimal sac. *Ophthalmology*, **87**, 476–482.

Pavilack, M. A. and Frueh, B. R. (1992). Thorough curettage in the treatment of chronic canaliculitis. *Arch. Ophthalmol.*, **110**, 200–202.

Pe'er, J. J., Stefanyszyn, M. D. and Hidayat, A. A. (1994). Nonepithelial tumours of the lacrimal sac. *Am. J. Ophthalmol.*, **118**, 650–658.

Welham, R. A. N. (1989). Lacrimal surgery. In *A Manual of Systematic Eyelid Surgery* (J. R. O. Collin, ed.), pp. 109–120. Churchill Livingstone.

Welham, R. A. N. and Bergin, D. J. (1985). Congenital lacrimal fistulas. *Arch. Ophthalmol.*, **103**, 545–548.

13

Surgery of canalicular obstruction

In the presence of a canalicular obstruction, routine DCR even with tubes will invariably fail. The choice of operation depends on the length of remaining patent canaliculus:

1. If there is more than 8 mm of one canaliculus present, a canaliculo-DCR may be performed.
2. If there is less than 8 mm of canaliculus, a DCR with bypass tube is required.

Canaliculo-DCR (CDCR)

Principle
An anastomosis is made between the end of one or both canaliculi and the nose, using the lacrimal sac if present as a bridging flap (Fig. 13.1).

Indications

1. An obstruction at or beyond 8 mm from the puncta of one or both canaliculi, but proximal to the common canaliculus at its junction with the sac.
2. Eight or more millimetres of patent canaliculus without any residual lacrimal sac in a patient having had a previous DCR.

Method

1. The incision is as for DCR (Fig. 13.2).
2. Place probes in the canaliculi, or a single probe if only one is present.
3. Raise the lateral skin flap towards the canthus and isolate the anterior limb of the medial canthal tendon (Fig. 13.3).
4. Divide the tendon near its periosteal insertion, and reflect it backwards (Fig. 13.4).

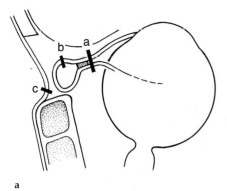

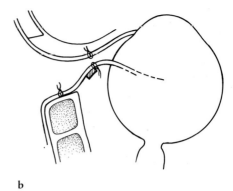

a

b

Fig. 13.1 a. Incisions for canaliculo-DCR. a = incision across most medial part of patent canaliculi; b = incision in anterior part of lacrimal sac; c = relatively posterior incision in nasal mucosa, to create large anterior flap.
b. The flaps sutured. The opened lacrimal sac acts as a bridge flap between the canaliculi and the posterior nasal mucosa.

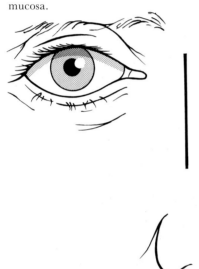

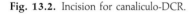

Fig. 13.2. Incision for canaliculo-DCR.

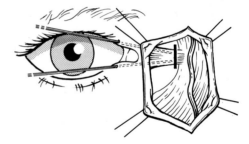

Fig. 13.3. The canthal tendon exposed and the canaliculi dissected wth probes within them.

5. With blunt dissection, separate the fibres of the orbicularis that are inserting in the region of the canthal tendon, to leave the probes within the medial canaliculi or lateral common canaliculus surrounded anteriorly (above and below) by only a thin collar of tissue.

6. Cut across the canaliculi at their most medial patent point (keeping the probes in place) (Fig. 13.5).

7. Proceed to elevate the periosteum and lacrimal sac (Fig. 13.6) and fashion the bony rhinostomy, making it big enough to allow a large anterior nasal mucosal flap to be fashioned (Fig. 13.7).

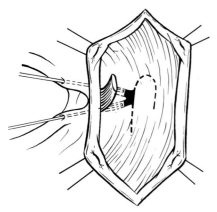

Fig. 13.4. The canthal tendon cut and reflected.

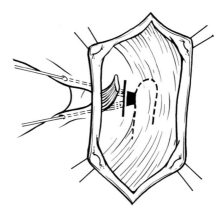

Fig. 13.5. An incision made across the most medial patent portion of the canaliculi.

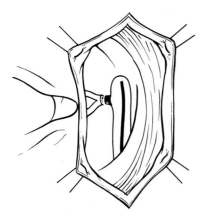

Fig. 13.6. Incision in the anterior part of the lacrimal sac.

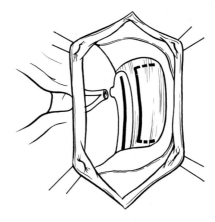

Fig. 13.7. Large anterior nasal mucosal flap fashioned.

8. Incise the lacrimal sac vertically at the point where the periosteum of the anterior lacrimal crest meets the sac (i.e. on its anterior border) (Fig. 13.6).

9. Incise the nasal mucosa to make a large anterior and a small posterior flap.

10. Swing the lacrimal sac open so that it forms a bridging flap between the canaliculi and the posterior nasal flap. Suture the sac to the posterior nasal flap with 6/0 chromic catgut sutures (Fig. 13.8).

11. Preplace several sutures in the end of the canaliculi, and suture them to the lacrimal sac flap posteriorly (Fig. 13.8).

12. Intubate the canaliculi, and pass the tubes into the nose and tie them (Fig. 13.9).

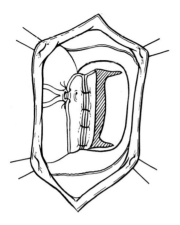

Fig. 13.8. The lacrimal sac opened and sutured as a bridge flap between the ends of the canaliculi and the posterior nasal mucosa.

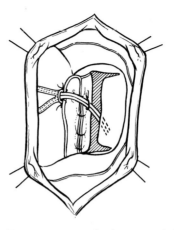

Fig. 13.9. Lacrimal tubing passed through the canaliculi into the nose.

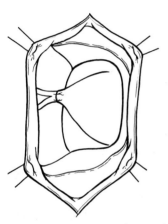

Fig. 13.10. Anterior nasal mucosal flap sutured across to the canaliculi.

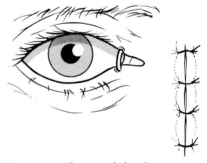

Fig. 13.11. The wound closed.

13. Suture the large anterior nasal flap to two preplaced sutures in the anterior wall of the ends of the canaliculi, so that the nasal flap is under some tension (Fig. 13.10).

14. Suture the skin (Fig. 13.11).

15. Remove the tubing after four months.

Complications

1. As for DCR.

2. Persistent watering with obstructed canaliculi, requiring a bypass tube.

DCR and bypass tube

If insufficient canaliculus is present for anastomosis into the nose, a bypass tube is required. The commonest bypass tube in use is made of pyrex glass (the Lester Jones tube). It acts as a conduit for tears from the conjunctival sac to the nose. As complications with the tube are common and long-term supervision is required, patients must be committed to regular review. Children may have surgery, provided they are mature enough to handle the tube in its day-to-day care.

Principle

A bypass tube is passed from the medial canthus through the soft tissues and the bony rhinostomy of a DCR into the nasal cavity.

Indications

1. Less than 8 mm of patent canaliculus.

2. A failed canaliculo-DCR.

3. A functional lacrimal obstruction not helped by a routine DCR (as in a complete facial palsy).

Method

1. Perform a standard DCR to the stage of suturing the posterior flaps.

2. Make sure the bony rhinostomy is sufficiently large inferiorly, so that the tube will not rest against bone.

3. At the medial canthus in the gap between lower lid and caruncle, pass a fine pointed guide wire through the soft tissues to emerge in the lateral wall of the opened lacrimal sac (Fig. 13.12a). It should pass in a medial and slightly inferior direction, roughly in the plane of the iris. Part or all of the caruncle may be removed to make room for the flanged end of the tube.

4. Pass a 1.5 or 2 mm trephine over the guide wire and remove a thin core of tissue between the canthus and the nose (Fig. 13.12b).

5. Remove the trephine and pass a tube over the guide wire and through the hole created by the trephine (Figs 13.13 and 13.14). Some force may be required to push it through, and a snug fit is desirable. The medial end of the tube should lie 2–3 mm clear of the nasal septum (Fig. 13.15), and the lateral end in a position that will allow free passage of tears in the lacrimal lake to enter the end of the tube.

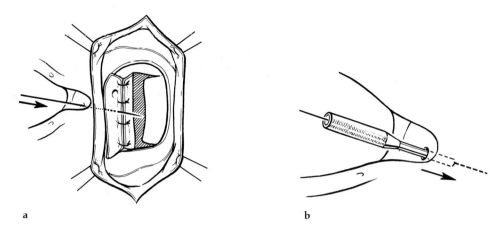

a   b

Fig. 13.12 a. Insertion of bypass tube. A sharp guide wire is passed from the medial canthus to emerge through the lateral wall of the lacrimal sac.
b. A small trephine passed over the guide wire.

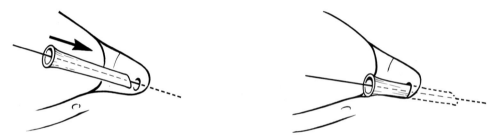

Figs 13.13 and 13.14. A bypass tube passed into position over the guide wire.

6. If the tube is of the wrong length, place a more appropriately sized tube and make a note of the length of the tube. If the tube does not sit neatly at the medial canthus and the caruncle is still present, its lower half may be excised to allow more space for the flanged end of the tube, or the whole caruncle may need to be excised.

7. If the anterior end of the middle turbinate is in the way of the tube, resect its anterior portion.

8. Suture the anterior flaps and close the skin (Fig. 13.16).

9. Anchor the tube in place by passing a 6/0 silk suture through the lid, around the tube twice and back out through the lid and over a bolster (Fig. 13.17). Remove the guide wire. Remove the anchoring suture at 10 to 14 days, when the tube will be more stable.

Complications

1. *Migration of the tube.* This is more common if the tube rests against

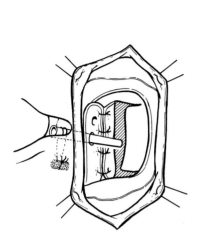

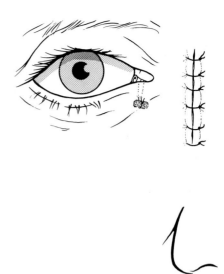

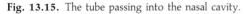

Fig. 13.15. The tube passing into the nasal cavity.

Fig. 13.16. The wound closed.

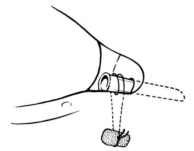

Fig. 13.17. The bypass tube sutured to the lid margin and tied over a bolster.

bone, and it may shift inwards or outwards. If the lateral end of the tube is buried in the soft tissues, reoperation will be required, with removal and repositioning of the tube. If the tube slips laterally, an early attempt is made to reposition it with local anaesthetic drops and infiltration if required. A plastic guide wire is inserted and an attempt to reinsert the tube is made. If this fails, formal reinsertion is required.

2. *Obstruction of the tube.* Occasionally, a mucus plug may block the tube. A fine plastic guide wire or lacrimal cannula will usually clear it. If necessary, the tube may be temporarily removed with a guide left in place, cleaned and reinserted. Another common source of obstruction is the plica of the conjunctiva, which may fold over the end of the tube. It may need to be excised or reduced in size, or the tube repositioned.

3. *Malposition of the tube.* If the tube is too far posterior and rests against the globe, or is not in a position to accept tears readily, it

should be removed. The track is allowed to close over and the tube is reinserted in a better position after a week or two.

4. *Granuloma formation.* Pyogenic granulomas may occur at the site of insertion. They are excised from their small base, and the base is cauterized.

Reinsertion of a bypass tube

Principle
A bypass tube is reinserted into the medial canthus where a DCR has previously been performed.

Indications

1. Migrated or malpositioned tube.
2. Lost tube.
3. A failed DCR with less than 8 mm of patent canaliculus.

Method

1. Pass a guide wire as above.
2. Using a nasal speculum and a head light, check that the guide wire is in the nose.
3. Trephine a fine core of tissue over the guide wire. Insert a tube of the previously noted length, or (if no tube has been previously placed) insert one that appears to be of appropriate length.
4. Inspect the position of the medial end of the tube in the nose to see that it is free within the nasal cavity and not up against the septum.
5. Secure the tube as above and remove the guide wire.

Repair of lacerated canaliculi

The commonest injury to the canaliculus is a laceration through the full thickness of the lower lid medial to the punctum (Fig. 13.18). This is most commonly a tractional tearing injury rather than a direct cut, as this is the weakest point of the lid. A similar injury may occur in the upper lid, or the two canaliculi may be divided.

Most patients are asymptomatic after repair of a single lacerated canaliculus, but many will also be asymptomatic after no formal repair.

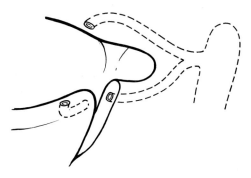

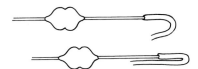

Fig. 13.18. Lacerated inferior canaliculus.

Fig. 13.19. Fine silicone tubing passed over the end of a fine lacrimal probe.

This merely indicates that a single canaliculus may be adequate to drain tears in most circumstances. In addition, a lacerated canaliculus that is not formally repaired will often form a fistula at the site of laceration, which may drain tears, but probably at a rate less than normal. These factors must be weighed against the risk of a surgical repair damaging the other (normal) canaliculus or the common canaliculus. If a method of repair is to be recommended, it should not have the potential to damage either the common canaliculus or the normal canaliculus.

REPAIR OF A SINGLE LACERATED CANALICULUS

Principle
A severed canaliculus is repaired and stented with fine silicone tubing, and the lid repaired in layers.

Method

1. Dilate the punctum and pass a probe to confirm the canaliculus is torn. Identify the medial end of the canaliculus – this is best done with a microscope. It is found near the posterior surface of the lid, just a few millimetres from the lid margin. If not found, fluorescein or air may be injected through the opposite canaliculus.

2. Using the same system as for intubation of the lacrimal system for congenital obstruction (a proprietary set of tubing or fine silicone tubing passed over a fine probe (Fig. 13.19) or blunt, long 25-gauge needle – see Chapter 11), pass the tubing through the proximal part of the system (Fig. 13.20) and then across the laceration, into the medial part of the canaliculus and into the sac (Fig. 13.21).

3. Pass it down the nasolacrimal duct as for an intubation and retrieve it from under the inferior turbinate (local anaesthetic packing will assist

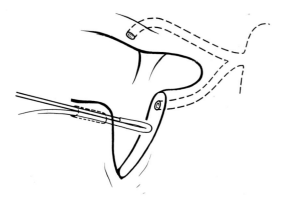

Fig. 13.20. Silicone tubing passed through the lateral portion of the lacerated canaliculus.

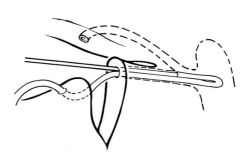

Fig. 13.21. Tubing passed into the medial portion of the canaliculus and into the sac.

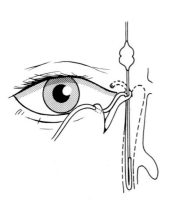

Fig. 13.22. The probe and tubing passed down the nasolacrimal duct and into the nose.

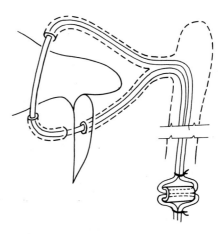

Fig. 13.23. Tubing passed through both canaliculi and secured in the nose beneath the inferior turbinate to prevent prolapse onto the eye.

this by shrinking the mucosa of the nose) (Fig. 13.22). Pass the other end of the tubing through the opposite canaliculus, nasolacrimal duct and nose, and secure the two ends as for congenital obstruction (Fig. 13.23).

4. If a repair is not possible, the medial end of the cut canaliculus can be intentionally marsupialized into the posterior surface of the lid.

5. Repair the canaliculus by preplacing two or three fine absorbable sutures (e.g. 8/0 vicryl) in the tissue surrounding the canaliculus (Fig. 13.24). Tie these, approximating the cut ends of the canaliculus.

6. Pulling on the tubing at the nostril approximates the ends of the canaliculi and facilitates this repair.

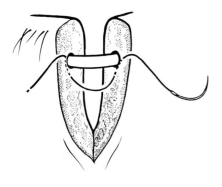

Fig. 13.24. Fine suture placed to approximate ends of canaliculi.

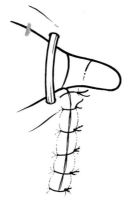

Fig. 13.25. Wound sutured in layers.

7. Repair the lid, taking care to re-approximate the posterior limb of the canthal tendon with a sufficiently posterior suture (Fig. 13.25).

8. Secure the tubing in the nose so that it cannot escape up the nasolacrimal duct. Remove it at three months.

REPAIR OF LACERATED UPPER AND LOWER CANALICULI

The prognosis of successful repair and lack of symptoms is considerably less in this case than for a single lacerated canaliculus. However, without repair, the patient will almost certainly have watering. The same system as described above can be utilized.

If the laceration is very medial, and in the region of the common canaliculus or lacrimal sac, a CDCR may be required to effect a repair. Opening the lacrimal sac allows retrograde probing of the canaliculi if identification of the cut ends is difficult.

Further reading

Henderson, P. N. (1985). A modified trephining technique for the insertion of Jones tube. *Arch. Ophthalmol.*, **103**, 1582–1585.

Rose, G. E. and Welham, R. A. N. (1991). Jones lacrimal canalicular bypass tubes: twenty-five years' experience. *Eye*, **5**, 13–19.

14

Endonasal lacrimal surgery

Endonasal lacrimal surgery has enjoyed a resurgence of interest over the past few years. It was abandoned many years ago because of its high rate of failure, but with newer endonasal instruments and endoscopes, the success rate has improved, although not reliably to the same level as can be achieved with standard external DCR. With time and refinement of techniques, the success rate may approach that of external DCR.

Primary endonasal DCR

Principle

An anastomosis is made between the lacrimal sac and the nose, operating from within the nasal cavity.

Indications

1. A desire to avoid the small external scar of a standard DCR.
2. Keloid scar formation.
3. Obstruction beyond the common canaliculus (endonasal DCR is likely to have a higher success when the lacrimal sac is normal or enlarged, as with a lacrimal mucocoele).

Advantages

1. Clear delineation of intranasal anatomy.
2. Ability to concurrently deal with nasal pathology such as adhesions and large middle turbinates that may obstruct the rhinostomy.
3. Avoidance of an external scar.

Disadvantages

1. Inability to deal adequately with common canalicular obstructions.
2. Inability to obtain mucosa-to-mucosa sutured anastomosis.
3. Higher failure rates.

4. Greater cost of instrumentation (endoscopes, endonasal instruments, lasers).

Method

General or local anaesthesia may be used.

1. Spray the nasal cavity with vasoconstrictive local anaesthetic and then pack with ribbon gauze soaked in an anaesthetic solution. (Direct injection can be made into the nasal mucosa at the site of surgery using a dental syringe.)

2. Pass a light-pipe (as used in vitreo-retinal surgery) along a canaliculus into the sac, to aid localization of the portion of the lateral nasal wall medial to the lacrimal sac. The light may then be visible in the lateral wall of the nose. The anatomic landmark for commencement of resection of nasal mucosa is a point just anterior to the uncinate process, and anterior to the anterior edge of the middle turbinate (Fig. 14.1a, b). An additional indicator is the convexity caused by the frontal process of the maxilla (externally, the anterior lacrimal crest), known as the agger nasi, which sometimes has an air cell between it and the lacrimal sac.

3. Use laser energy (delivered by fibreoptic) or diathermy to ablate the mucosa overlying the lacrimal sac, or remove it with endonasal forceps after incision with a sickle knife (Fig. 14.2a).

4. Remove the bone between the lacrimal sac and the nose by use of a high-energy laser, high-speed burr or rongeurs (Fig. 14.2b). Pay attention to removal of some of the thicker bone of the anterior lacrimal crest, and all the bone between the sac and upper

Fig. 14.1 a. The lateral wall of the nose. a = the agger nasi; b = middle turbinate; c = inferior turbinate; d = nasal vestibule.
b. The lateral wall of the nose to show the position of the lacrimal sac and nasolacrimal duct. a = lacrimal sac.

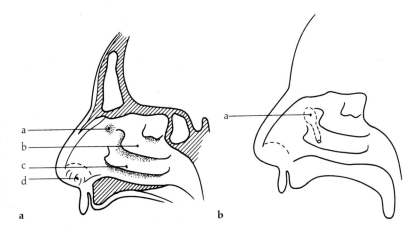

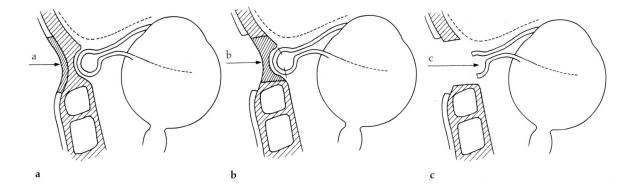

Fig. 14.2. Axial section of the lateral nasal wall and lacrimal sac. a = area of nasal mucosa to be removed; b = area of bone to be removed; c = lacrimal sac opened and its medial wall excised.

nasolacrimal duct and the nose. If an ethmoidal air cell is encountered, it should also be removed.

5. The medial wall of the lacrimal sac should now be visible. Tent it up with the light pipe or a lacrimal probe. Make a vertical incision in the sac, and remove the mucosa of the medial wall of the sac using laser or forceps (Fig. 14.2c).

6. Pass silicone tubing through the lacrimal system and tie the two ends to avoid prolapse onto the eye, or pass a short sleeve of larger tubing over the two ends and advance it towards the lacrimal sac. Take care to avoid making the loop of tubing too tight, as this may cause cheese-wiring of the canaliculi.

7. Antimetabolites such as mitomycin C may be placed on the rhinostomy site to diminish postoperative scarring, and hopefully to improve success rates.

8. Postoperatively, inspect the rhinostomy at weekly intervals for several weeks and remove any crusts or debris.

9. Remove the silicone tubing after two to three months.

Complications

1. Failure due to closure of the rhinostomy or occlusion of the common canaliculus.

2. Primary or secondary haemorrhage.

3. Prolapse of orbital fat into the wound if the periorbita behind the lacrimal sac is traumatized.

Secondary endonasal DCR

Indications

1. Failed external or endonasal DCR.

2. Patency of the canaliculi and common canaliculus.

3. Intranasal pathology such as adhesions.

Method
Anaesthesia and preparation are the same as for primary endonasal DCR.

1. Pass a probe along one canaliculus as far as possible.

2. Inspect the nose using the endoscope, and identify the site of the previous rhinostomy.

3. Remove the middle turbinate or any adhesions, if present, at the rhinostomy.

4. Remove the mucosa and scar tissue overlying the end of the probe using laser, diathermy or forceps, until the probe appears in the nose. Enlarge the opening so that the whole of the lacrimal sac is visible.

5. Antimetabolites may be applied to the re-opened rhinostomy.

6. Pass silicone tubing and secure it as for primary endonasal DCR.

7. Inspect and clean the rhinostomy at weekly intervals for several weeks.

8. Remove the silicone tubing after three months.

Complications
These are the same as for primary endonasal DCR.

Endonasal-assisted insertion of bypass tube

Lester Jones bypass tubes may be inserted as described in Chapter 13, and the position within the nasal cavity checked with the aid of an endoscope. A speculum and head light may be used, but the view will be more magnified and unobstructed with an endoscope. Another advantage is the ability to deal with a middle turbinate that sits at the desired position of the tube, or with other nasal pathology that may reduce the successful placement of the tube.

Further reading

Bartley, G. B. (1994). The pros and cons of laser dacryocystorhinostomy. *Am. J. Ophthalmol.,* **117**, 103–106.

Boush, G. B., Lemke, B. N. and Dortzbach, R. K. (1994). Results of endonasal laser-assisted dacryocystorhinostomy. *Ophthalmology,* **101**, 955–959.

Whittet, H. B., Shun-Shin, G. A. and Awdry, P. (1993). Functional endoscopic transnasal dacryocystorhinostomy. *Eye,* **7**, 545–549.

Index